Labor Pains and Birth Stories

Essays on Pregnancy, Childbirth, and Becoming a Parent

edited by Jessica Powers

CATALYST BOOK PRESS

San Bruno, California

Acknowledgements

"On the Day Sage was Born" by Annalysa Lovos was originally published in *Mothering Magazine.*

Catalyst Book Press ISBN 978-0-9802081-1-5
Library of Congress Control Number (LCCN) 2008908477

To order additional copies of the book, contact Catalyst Book Press
www.catalystbookpress.com, info@catalystbookpress.com

I would like to thank Kathy McInnis for her excellent book cover, Tania Pryputniewicz for her great cover image and for copy-editing, Erik Powers for copy-editing, and Dennis and Becky Powers for being great parents for 30-plus years.

This book is dedicated to my best friend Tabitha Spitzer.

Table of Contents

Table of Contents
continued

Introduction

I am what you might call a birth story aggregator. I did not start out doing this for fun, or science, or prurient interests. Rather, I began collecting birth stories of various vintages and cultural orientations for perspective.

I had my own birth story, an unexpected and perhaps unnecessary cesarean, but I had no idea whether that ordeal should be considered good, bad or somewhere in between. Was I lucky or supremely unlucky? I needed to know how 12 hours of labor, followed by 20 minutes or so in the operating room that produced a perfectly healthy baby being lifted out of an incision in my abdomen, and culminating in months of painful recuperation, compared and contrasted with other women's experiences

First, I looked to the women in my own family, whose tales were, well, a panoply of horrors. Then I cast the net to include my friends, colleagues, and a few others whom I sort of knew on a first-name basis—celebrities. Hm. Then, I began to dig a bit deeper, into historical accounts, old magazines, newspapers, antique diaries, books chock full of birth practices from far off lands.

What I learned was that every generation and every culture has its own way of giving birth. That is the story writ large. But I also learned that every woman, for every birth, has a unique story to tell. Many such tales hook us with those familiar words "I went into labor at…" Yet it is the vast unknown between such an opening and the finale ("It's a boy!") that almost anyone will stop and listen to—or read about. We share these stories because giving birth is an important rite of passage. We share these stories because, on occasion, they serve as cautionary tales and there is therapy in retelling. And we share these stories because we are proud and can't help but spread the joy.

This anthology is a white-knuckle ride through vastly different experiences, writing styles and emotions. Through these twists and turns my perspective lurched back and forth several times, settling somewhere at the intersection of bitter and sweet. I hope you enjoy this collection as much as I did.

Tina Cassidy, Author of *Birth: The Surprising History of How We Are Born*
Boston
2008

1

The Baby Project

Amy Parker

I think every girl who knows she wants to grow up and have kids fantasizes about being pregnant and giving birth. *How does it feel to be pregnant? How will I look? What happens in a delivery room? What will I have, a boy or a girl?* I was no different than any other little girl imagining the wonders of pregnancy and birth... except I forgot to factor my diabetes into my fantasy. Never did I imagine as a 19-year-old in art school that I would be told I could not do something. All my life I was told, "If you can dream it, you can do it."

My "dream" was to be pregnant, to have children. I dreamed of a ceramics studio at my home, and carting a baby around in a sling carrier on my back as I threw bowls and prepared for shows, like the images I had seen of indigenous women of South America. I never ever dreamed that my doctor would tell me, "It's not a good idea for you to get pregnant. Your kidneys are just too weak...why don't you just adopt?"

First of all, no doctor on this earth should have a portrait in his office of himself, flanked by his wife, four children in matching outfits, and their golden retriever on the beach while telling a young woman that having children is just not going to happen. Second of all, the term "just adopt" should be wiped from the English language altogether. Families who adopt do not "just" do anything. As my husband and I found out, families who "just adopt" are the ones who are willing to put themselves under a microscope for any inspector, just for the approval of becoming parents.

After my husband and I were officially married, we talked about babies morning, noon and night. How would we get one? Where do we start? Why can those people have five kids and complain about not having a boy after having four girls, when all we wanted was one baby? After mourning the loss of the idea of having a child with my husband's buggy blue eyes and my sense of humor, we got used to the idea of our child not looking like us…and celebrated the idea of being able to call ourselves fortunate enough to adopt a child. We knew people who said things like, "I couldn't raise a child that wasn't biologically mine." It made us laugh inside because we knew we were the lucky ones. We were the family who was open to raising our children with diversity, understanding, and respect for all people.

But as we dove into the adoption process head first, my little sister, 20 years old at the time, said to us, "Hey, if you are interested, I would love to carry a baby for you. I've researched it and I would be glad to help in any way I can."

Floored by this offer, my husband and I came to a screeching halt. Wait, you mean we could have a biological child? What about respect and diversity? What about being the lucky ones? What about "just adopt"??

We decided that we had nothing to lose. After all, there weren't any rules about adopting after we had a biological babe, right? We had six months to sit on this idea while we waited for my sister to graduate from college. My sister submerged herself so deeply into what we called "the baby project" that she dedicated her final semester in undergrad, with a major in Sociology and a minor in Women's Studies, to completing a research paper on gestational surrogacy that won her awards at her college.

That fall, we made our first visit to a fertility clinic. We sat there, hopeful sponges, ready for any information that was going to let us know that we would indeed become parents someday, and hopefully, someday soon. We got started right away with all the shots, and pills, and calendars, and sonograms, et cetera. We were psyched. The day of my egg retrieval came along and we hoped to hear that everything was "a go." Turns out my eggs weren't mature and after retrieving 23 eggs out of my enormous ovaries, through my sore uterus wall, only two embryos were viable. My sister, husband and I joked about the pornography selection at the hospital and the poor guy who had to stand outside of the collection room on the day of the egg retrieval. We named the two embryos "Zelda and Froggy" after F. Scott Fitzgerald's wife and character Froggy Parker.

Two weeks passed, and we had ourselves a negative pregnancy test.

My poor sister had to sit in her room alone while I lay in bed, furious that I was not being given a chance. Where was my control? Why wasn't I in control? After a few days of mourning, we decided, "Let's give it another go." I mean, we threw a few grand at the doctor already, what was a few more?

Let us just put it this way: second verse, same as the first, except this time I was angry. I knew people who had tried IVF many times and kept on going until they found success, but how the heck did they do it? How were these people so strong? I was running out of strength.

It was the day we got our second negative pregnancy test back that we decided to contact an adoption attorney and pursue a domestic adoption. I needed a baby with the umbilical cord raisin thingy. I needed to hear the shrill sounds of a newborn and smell that sweet shampoo head. I wanted to lay with the baby and listen to wee little goat sounds every time the baby grunted or moved. A private, domestic adoption seemed to be the route we needed to take.

When I called the adoption attorney on a cool, spring, Monday morning, he asked, "Well, how soon do you want a baby?"

When people ask you questions such as this, there is not a correct answer. I thought to myself, "Uuhh, YESTERDAY!" Clearly, that was not the correct answer. So I said, in my most educated voice, just as Adoptions for Dummies taught me, "As long as it takes for our home study to be completed and whenever there is a baby available, I guess."

With an appreciative laugh, the voice on the other end of the phone said, "If you hurry up and get to my office, there will be a baby available in two weeks, but time is of the essence, and you have a lot of paperwork to fill out."

I hung up the phone and urped a little. Then I said to my husband, who was showering, "We could have a baby in two weeks. Is that okay?" It was as if I was checking his schedule to make dinner plans with friends.

The curtain pulled slowly away from the wall and steam poured out and fogged up my glasses. He was pale, but smiling.

I said, "Does this feel right?"

He said, "Ummm, yeah?…but why does it need to be so fast?"

The family giving their baby up for adoption already had six children and could not afford a seventh. I was on the fence with how I should feel about, and for, this baby. How awful would it feel to be the one "they could not afford"? But I hauled over to the attorney's office to fill out all the forms. The attorney in Florida, where the adoption was going to take place, reported that the family was "uncomfortable" with my husband's age; they thought he was too young. The birth father was 31 and my husband was only going on 30. My husband was clearly too young. What the?? Clearly.

As fast as the attorney broke it to me that "It isn't going to work out with that baby," she whipped out another profile of another pregnant woman in a pinch—just like a breeder explains that the pick of the litter is already sold, but this other one has a better temperament. As I picked my heart up off of the floor, she handed me the profile of a woman I'll call Sara. Sara was single, had three children, and seemed so sad in the picture in her birthmother profile. I called my husband and talked over the profile with him. She was clean and sober. She had a job and she had a high-school education. She was a star on her high-school swim team. She just ran into tough times: a sticky divorce and a boyfriend who took off when he heard she was pregnant. My husband and I agreed that the situation was sad, but hopefully we could all work together and make for a happier situation. Sara did not have custody of her children due to a grand theft charge, but she was going to court after the baby was born to get custody of her three children back.

Sara needed money to help pay her rent, phone, electricity, gas, and medical bills. We gladly paid all of those expenses and offered to get her counseling and maternity clothes. We met Sara three weeks later. She was quiet and sweet. She was glad to hear that we had big families and lots of crazy kids in our lives. She was thrilled to hear that I grew up on a farm and that I visited the farm almost weekly to see my family. She chit-chatted with us about our dogs and our home. She showed interest in the town in which we lived. She wondered if we preferred a boy or a girl. Sara gave me a huge hug and lifted her shirt to show me her beautiful round belly. Sara said to me, "Would you be comfortable in the delivery room with me? I'm scared to deliver the baby alone and I don't want the baby ever to see my face. You will be the baby's mother, and the baby needs to only see you." I got chills.

She was due the first week in September. It was April. We only had a few months to get ready but the way I saw it, it was just a shorter pregnancy for us. Sara even sent us sonogram pictures, sonogram pictures I carried around, proudly showing off to all my friends and family. By the looks of it, the baby in the sonogram picture was a beautiful girl. She had a beautiful profile and dainty hands. My friends swore there was a penis between the legs but I was not convinced. We did not know the gender of the babe, but we decided on a name: Betty Jeanne. We never could decide on a boy's name. We were so certain about Betty Jeanne that a boy's name never felt right.

In August, we got news that Sara needed more money to help pay for medication for gestational diabetes. I all of a sudden felt a connection. This woman had the very disease that kept me from giving birth to a baby. We quickly sent a check. At the end of August, we started to worry that Sara would go into labor and be alone. We made plans to stay at my aunt and uncle's place in Florida. They insisted that we stay at their place. We understood all the rules and regulations of their gated community and we were finally comfortable with the idea of going to Florida as a couple and returning home as a family.

I was sort of sad that no one wanted to throw me a big baby shower with all the geeky baby booty decorations and pink and blue flowers. I really wanted to register for cool baby clothes and this neat bouncy seat I saw on an alternative baby website. But there was this looming tone that the adoption could fall through and we would be "stuck" with all this baby junk, a constant reminder that we were childless. So instead of a shower, we planned on having a big party when we returned home from Florida with our bundle.

Right before our trip, I packed a big black duffle bag with cloth diapers, hooded towels, onesies, little yellow socks, a soft organic cotton blanket, a rented breast pump (because I was going to nurse this baby if it was the last thing I did, and I had all the alternative literature to prove that it could be done), and a portable co-sleeper. We packed it all up and called my aunt and uncle to let them know that we had made arrangements to fly to Florida and that we would be using their house.

We received a phone call from my aunt the night before we left for Florida. She said, "We are not comfortable with you staying at our place until after the baby is born. We didn't offer you that place as a free place to stay. Your uncle takes great pride in that home and we didn't think you would take advantage. Your uncle's own kids haven't ever stayed in that house. You should feel honored that he even offered."

I felt like a wet noodle after I hung up the phone. My husband tried to understand through my sobs. We just could not understand why they would insist and then renege the offer. It sucked. So the weekend before Labor Day, we scrambled to find a place to stay indefinitely while all the adoption process was finalized. It was possible that we could be there for more than a few weeks.

We finally found a room at an extended stay hotel. We were set. We were nauseous, but we were set. We arrived in Florida on a beautiful summer day. We found the hotel. I nested for a few hours. We went to the grocery store and bought enough food to feed a starving third world country, went back to the place, had a little happy hour, and showered. We found a Houston's restaurant in town. We loved the Houston's back home, so this did the trick. While we were waiting for our appetizer, the appetizer I used to crave weekly, I had a major anxiety attack. I mean I was freaking out. All I wanted to do was throw up all over the table. I had to go. I had to get out of there. I needed to forget the whole thing and go home: back to my bed, back to my friends, back to my dogs. Home. This place was not home; it was Hell. We left the restaurant and went back to the hotel. I took a warm shower, and put in a call to my therapist.

We contacted the adoption attorney the next day and gave him all of our contact information. Every time the phone rang, we ran so fast to pick it up, our skeletons left our skin. The last phone call I remember was from our adoption attorney. Sara already had the baby and was keeping "her." Sara apologized in a letter. She said she "couldn't bear to part with a baby girl." I whole-heartedly believed that that was honestly how she felt, and that she would make do. People do that. People survive. My husband believed that the 20 grand we shelled out to "help" Sara was a ploy to feed her boyfriend's drug habit. We returned to our home—quiet, empty, and sad.

We received phone calls from friends and family, offering to listen and help. My aunt who offered the use of her house in Florida and then took back the offer must have called five times between the days of Rosh Hashanah and Yom Kippur. In hindsight, she was probably being a caring aunt. Back then, we believed that all she wanted was our forgiveness to avoid God's wrath. For months, I was a mess. For months, my husband tried to understand. I stopped eating. Food made me sick. My husband would say, "Ugh! Eat already. Remember you used to like food?!" I just could not eat. I was thrilled when I felt the teeniest bit hungry.

After all the holidays were over, we started to mention possibly adopting a baby from China. We could definitely get a baby from China. You hardly ever hear of a birth mother keeping her baby in China. We were safe in China. We jumped in headfirst again. We were all about China: China this and China that. We watched shows about China, and read stories about China. "Let's get this homestudy goin'!" We did it all. The dossier was almost done. The last thing we had to do was have a portrait taken of the both of us in a fun activity (while wearing pants, not shorts), happy and together. I have got to say, I seemed happy, but sometimes I felt sad for the baby we would adopt. What about her poor mom who was forced to abandon her sweet baby girl on the steps of a church or school? We would not be able to ever trace her parents. I tried to figure out ways to build up a history for her that involved us and not her biological parents but still, there was an emptiness that I felt responsible to fill. After all, I was feeling empty too. Maybe we could in some way feel, without being too Jerry Maguire, "complete."

We were almost there. We were feeling good. Then, our adoption attorney said, "Have you thought about trying egg donation through another fertility clinic? One of my good friends is the head of the program at another fertility center." We let her make us an appointment. I mean, after all, when your people know people it never hurts, plus we had nothing to lose, we were going to China.

We went to the new clinic. We were wooed with bells and whistles, fancy waiting room furniture and exotic travel magazines. We spoke with the head doctor. We discussed getting donor eggs and using my husband's sperm, so we would be safe. We would have legal rights if one of us was a biological parent. The doctor looked at our charts and said, "I don't think you'll need donor eggs. I think I can make this work. I don't want to force you into something you don't feel up to doing and of course I would like to be your hero, but I do honestly think I can do this. I've made it happen for other women with diabetes." Ohhhh, he was fantastic: a Paul Simon look alike with a South African accent.

My heart jumped. But I had that internal conflict. One voice was yelling, "Run away from the light, you can't go through this again, you just started feeling hungry again!!!" The other voice in my head was a Nike commercial: "Just do it!! You can do it…you can do it…. Do it!"

After I realized that I was probably making funny faces while everyone looked at me, my husband and I spoke in private. We would do it, but I did not want my sister to carry. She had already taken a year and a half out of her life for us. She was finally doing stuff for herself. The doctor understood, but he said, "Don't make the choice for her. I've seen families ripped apart because of assumptions. Ask her. She has the right to make her own choices."

Oh jeez, where did this guy come from? He was so wise, and that accent!! I caught myself staring. I blinked twice and said, "Okay, we'll give her a call and let you know."

My sister had to think about it. It was not something that she quickly agreed to do. She needed her own space. She needed to have a job. She needed to have her own life. After awhile, however, she called back and said, "Okay, let's do this. I started this baby project, and I'm going to finish it. I want the relationship with the baby." So we jumped on it. We got all psyched as we had done before. We got all hormonal and bitchy. We laughed about pornography in "the little room." We said the word "sperm" so much, we snorted drinks out of our noses, laughing so hard. We laughed. We cried. We trudged on and on and on. I was not as stressed this time, because I knew if it did not work, we had a baby in China waiting for us, hypothetically of course, since we never actually handed in our dossier. If it did work, we would have two babies. We would have one baby with blue eyes and one baby with Chinese eyes.

The Baby Project

The day came for the ol' egg retrieval. It went well. The embryos formed. We picked out the two best quality embryos and transferred them into my sister's primed uterine wall. We all watched and clapped. We joked and said, "Was it as good for you as it was for me??" We went home. My sister lay on the couch with her hips elevated for two days.

My hormones were raging. *Why is she in that position? Why aren't I allowed to be her? Why isn't there any place for me to sit? Why can't we have what I want for dinner? Why is my sister so grumpy?* Ugh! I had to get out of there. Again I left the scene and had a temper tantrum in private that would make a two-year-old jealous. I was self centered and bitchy. After all, she was doing this for me.

Luckily, I snapped out of it after the hormones eased up, and started getting myself ready for pregnancy test day.

The day rolled around. My sister and I went to the clinic. She got her blood drawn and we decided that we needed to shop. I mean, shop like we had any money left to burn. So, we went to our favorite store, Anthropologie. She was having a ball. I was having a heart attack. My good friend, who was now also my sister's boyfriend, tagged along. He was acting rather seriously. His typical serious attitude always made me snicker, but this time I wished he would make a joke or something. My cell phone rang in the store. After flipping it in the air a hundred times, just like a cartoon character, I answered it nervously. The call was from our IVF nurse. She said very stoically, "We have your test results. Why don't you come to the office and we can discuss your options?" I knew it was bad. I was shaking. I said, "Let's roll," and made that hand sign as if I was an air traffic control officer. My sister's beau / my friend sped up the highway so fast that I said, "Um, can we slow down? I'm dying to know the results, not die in a car accident."

My husband met us at the clinic. We were ushered into a private room and the door was closed. We stood nervously holding hands. Our nurse walked in and said, "Congratulations!! We did it!" My knees buckled. I cried hysterically. We all hugged, and jumped around like a bunch of schoolgirls when a hottie walks by. Oh wow. We were psyched.

Then our nurse said, "But there's bad news." There was the familiar needle on the record. She added, "The beta cell count is very high." There should be 100 cells per embryo. My sister's beta count was currently 400. We all silently did the math. Was it possible that our two embryos not only took, both of them divided? Dear God, it was all or nothing with us. Our nurse said, "See, the thing is, it's safer to not carry a high number of multiples, so if we see in a sonogram in two weeks that there are more than three embryos, you might want to talk selective reduction." Wait, like an abortion? Did she say reduction? That word was worse than cussing.

I looked at my sister. She was making a major sad face. So I pulled this out of my ass: "Hey, not to worry, if there's a reason to worry after we know what's really happening then we worry, but for now, let's be excited."

Two weeks later, we returned to the fertility center for the sonogram we had waited to do for four years now. We watched the sonogram tech smear that cold jelly all over my sister's flat stomach. The doctor said, "There's one...and there's one. I don't see any more...looks like a two-fer." There was a collective sigh.

It was wonderful. But why did we still feel so uncertain? Why did I keep thinking that something bad was going happen? We were ushered into a waiting room and handed info on obstetricians and drug protocols, and the number for the area Mothers of Multiples club.

We were glad. We were glad pretty much all the time after that. When I say pretty much all the time, I mean most of the time for my husband and half of the time for me. Again, I was in selfish mode. They were my babies. Why couldn't I carry them? As my sister threw up for six months, I felt bad because she was feeling rotten but I wanted to feel rotten, too. I wanted maternity clothes and people rubbing my round belly. I wanted people to ask me when my baby was due.

I drove two hours each day to inject hormones into my sister's tender butt. She did it with a smile on her face. I took her out to dinner a lot. She was a real trooper. I sucked at being appreciative. I loved her more than anything, but my jealousy was eating me up. I missed out on most of our pregnancy being jealous until one day, while we were at my parents' place at the beach, my sister said, "Baby A is kicking. Wanna feel?" I placed my right hand on her big belly and felt the most miraculous thing—the foot of my baby kick the center of my hand. It really did feel like a goldfish in a plastic bag. It hit me: we were going to have a family in a few months and we had so much to learn.

During our visits to the OB and sonogram lab, we always stood out. Were we an adoptive mom and a birth mother? Were we lesbians? What was our deal? We explained it to so many people so many times: "She's my oven. I'm the biological mother." We joked about having a t-shirt made with the top ten questions gestational carriers hear with answers on the back. Answers like: "No, I'm just the oven, she's the mom"; "Yes, like Phoebe on Friends"; "No, I didn't sleep with my brother-in-law"; "Yes, I know I have to give them away after they are born"; and "No, I do not want to keep them."

We really needed that t-shirt one day at a visit to the sonogram lab. I asked the sonogram technician if that day was the day we could find out the gender of the babies because we did not want to know. The tech's response: "It doesn't matter what you want to know or don't want to know, I only care about my patient."

My whole body sagged. I think my heart skipped a beat. My eyes immediately welled up. I didn't matter. I was no more part of this project than any other member of my family. I didn't feel them every day. I wasn't growing them. I even listened to my mother talk about my "poor" sister and how she was feeling so sick all the time. I knew that I was wrong for feeling angry, but sometimes I just needed to be a crank.

My sister's response to this sonogram tech was golden. She said, "Um, you should care. She's the biological mother. I want whatever she wants."

I perked up. My sister said it. Straight up.

The tech looked at her chart and said, "I'm sorry, I didn't see that in the chart."

That day will stick with me forever.

They were 12 weeks away, but we were ready. We had clothes, four names picked out, a crib. (Only one, because they would co-bed if it was the last thing I did.) On October 6, the four of us plus two in utero went out to dinner together. We returned to my sister's house and hung out until it got late and we needed to get a move on. We laughed and talked and watched my sister's stomach get tight. She would say, "Oh, these darn Braxton-Hicks contractions!"

We woke up when the phone rang at about 8 a.m. on October 7th. I heard my sister say, "I started to feel 'weird' this morning, so I called my OB. He told me that it was normal to have contractions at the end of the second trimester, especially with multiples. I explained that I could time the contractions and he said, 'Go to the ER. Have them hook you up to a monitor.' So we are on our way." My husband and I threw on some clothes. I remember that sinking feeling in my gut and in my brain. I remember sitting on my hands so they would hurt more than my head. I remember saying, "It's too early. I don't want them to have to struggle." My husband and I talked about who knows what to pass the time. Most of what was said was, "Why does this stuff happen to us?" about 1000 different ways.

We got to the hospital, we explained who we were, and we were directed to the triage area of the labor and delivery ward. My sister looked rough, but not rough like she was in pain, rough like she was scared. The nurse examined my sister and said that everything looked okay. A doctor came in and did the final evaluation and all of a sudden things went awry. My sister had dilated to two centimeters in a matter of minutes. A team of nurses and doctors whisked her into a private room. I followed close so I did not miss a beat. I was shushed out of the room so they could catheterize my sister and start her on a magnesium drip. I stood in the hallway with my husband, crying. "It's too early. They're too little."

Our mom showed up less than an hour later, worried times two. What strength she had to stand in a hospital room, watching her youngest daughter lay motionless in a hospital bed, while the other daughter stood at her sister's bedside as a spectator to her own children's struggle. Mom did a great job making sure everyone in our family knew what was happening and making sure arrangements were being made for everything under the sun at home and in the hospital.

About 20 minutes after my sister was admitted into the hospital, a nurse walked up to us and asked us if we would fill out these forms for the morgue and if we wanted a priest to visit my sister and bless the babies after they were born. Here's where it gets a little confusing. My husband and I are interfaith but really agnostic. Let me tell you, my belief in God at that moment was nil. I stood there a little teary. What if I was wrong, and we did not bless the babes and we punished them because of our lack of faith and distrust of organized religion? Clearly, we were in a pinch, but decided to waive the priest visit. I was uncomfortable with any clergy at that moment, especially a priest, since neither of us is Catholic. I asked myself a jillion times, "Are we wrong? And whoa, what's this about a morgue?" Holy crap, this was serious.

On the charts, my sister was 27 weeks. On our charts, she was too early for our comfort. My amazing sister lay motionless for three days. The only time she moved was to throw up into a bedpan. I patted her head with a freezing cold washcloth, since one of the side effects of magnesium is to feel extremely hot. We helped her do something we coined "the swish and spit." Because magnesium sulfate relaxes every muscle in the body, my sister could not swallow, although her mouth was extremely dry. Her eyes had a tough time blinking. My husband and I sat vigil at her bedside, swapping shifts for sleep breaks.

Finally, the contractions slowed down enough for her to stop the magnesium and get on a tributeline drip. All was well. My sister was sitting up. The babies were growing away in her belly. We were happy. It was a beautiful day outside. Life was good. So….My husband went back to work. We were told that my sister was going to be moved to a mother-baby ward on bed rest for the rest of her pregnancy. All we needed was to be discharged by the OB and we were going to roll to a more comfortable room.

The doctor came in to do the exam at about two in the afternoon. Her little head popped up from under my sister's legs and said, "You can't move. You're dilated to four centimeters." All of a sudden, three nurses rushed into the room wielding IV fluids and syringes. The nurse said to us, "We have to put you back on Magnesium."

I could see my sister's body sink. I could not possibly understand how magnesium felt but I knew she was tired of all of this. She was finally feeling a little better after the first hit of magnesium. She could finally eat jello and drink chicken broth!

Then the OB walked in and said, "No magnesium, these babies are ready to come out."

The perinatologist flew in and said, "Mag."

The neonatologist said, "Magnesium! I can't believe you would consider not giving her magnesium!"

Everyone was staring at my sister. I spoke to all of the doctors separately and all of them had a different opinion. The OB said, "No mag; mag makes babies lethargic at birth, and we need these babies to be angry and strong." The perinatologist and neonatoligist said, "27 ½ weeks is too early, they are not ready."

I decided that since the doctors could not make up their minds, it was time to ask my sister how she felt. My sister was hesitant. She trusted her OB and felt that her doctor would not lead her down the wrong path. We were so confused so she opted to take the magnesium one more time. She said that we had gotten this far and she would hate to make a bad decision selfishly. As my husband sped back to the hospital, I sat with my sister and we talked quietly about baby names and how much fun twins were going to be.

The magnesium did not stop the contractions this time. The contractions were coming every two minutes or so. My sister dilated from four centimeters to eight centimeters in less than an hour. It was time.

We were scared, but there was no time for fear. My husband ran into the room, winded and scared. We were told that only one person could be in the room with my sister. It was awkward, but my husband, being as awesome as ever, said, "You go." I spoke with the OB one last time. She was on the phone this time, as she had to run and check on another patient. I asked her if this was really going to be okay. She said to me, "Amy, in my country (India) there is a saying that goes like this: The elephant has passed, only the tail remains."

I thought to myself, "Wow, she's so wise. Things are going to be just fine." It was that OB's calming voice and her humanity that made me understand that this was for real and everything would work out just fine.

A nurse busted into the supply closet where I was on the phone and threw some scrubs at me, saying, "Put these on and meet us in the OR." I sized the men's XXXL scrubs up to my five-foot-two frame and sort of giggled but I did not have any other options. I put the paper scrubs on and walked into our room. I sighed and saw three sets of eyes staring at me. My husband hugged and kissed me. I cannot remember what he said now, but I'm sure it was encouraging with a hint of apprehension and realism. My mom said something like, "This is it," and kissed me.

I walked into the room where my sister was given an epidural. She was getting situated on the operating table in preparation for a c-section. "Baby A" was transverse, so a c-section was our only option. I nervously sat on a stool and held her hand. We said our favorite cheer from high-school: we had loved to poke fun at the cheerleaders back in the day. "B-E A-G-G-R-E-S-S-I-V-E...be aggressive, be, be aggressive, yay! Goooo babies!!!" The studly anesthesiologist watched from behind us, probably thinking we were immature. So, trying to make light of a profound experience, we sat there with forced smiles for what seemed like hours.

In about three or four minutes, a sound erupted above the bells and whistles of the OR. This sound was exactly like this: a kitten mewing. This wee little sound mewed five or six times and was quiet for a few seconds. We were told that preemies use up all of their energy with the first scream so to expect the babies to be put on ventilators to help save their energy. There was a bunch of hustling behind the big blue tarp, hiding the most important moment of our lives, but then we heard that kitten sound again and the chills came back. I heard a nurse say, "It's a girl," very quietly. As the nurses scurried around the OR, I overheard the OB talking about "baby B's" arm placement. She said, "It's beautiful, look at these beautiful fingers, look at the baby's arm, so graceful, absolutely beautiful." I was so taken by this statement. There she was, just doing her job, a job she's been doing for more than 20 years, and she was still amazed by the miracle of birth and the beauty of a newborn child. I still get chills when I think of that moment.

"Baby B" was delivered a minute after "Baby A." I heard a voice say, "It's a boy." The shrill mewing coming from behind that tarp made me realize that this was the very reason I was put on this earth and I hadn't even seen the kids yet. I was just happy to finally hear them. For years, I had practiced saying in the bathroom mirror, "Hi, I've been waiting for so long to meet you. I'm your mommy. I love you so much." I was prepped and ready. I bawled along with my sister. I told her that my husband and I had decided that if the babies were boy-girl twins, the girl's middle name would be my sister's first name, which is Susan.

A nurse walked over with what we now call a "baby burrito" and said, "Here's the boy." He was a little mentch. All scrunched up. I was ready to say what I had practiced all those years, "Hi, I'm your mommy, etc…" but "You look just like your grandfather!" blurted out of me. I stopped myself, surprised. Oh man! I had messed up already! Well, I guess I was just being the master of the obvious and my brain felt like speaking the truth. Baby B still looks like his grandfather sometimes, but his appearance flip-flops between both of his grandfathers. If baby B grew a beard, he would be the spittin' image of my dad. After all was done in the delivery room, I walked back to the room where my husband, my mom, and my sister's boyfriend waited to hear the news.

This was the biggest news of my life. This is also the single most regrettable moment of my life—the one thing I would take back. Instead of pulling my husband out into the hall, or to the side, so we could celebrate as husband and wife, I busted into the room and said, with no regard to my husband's feelings, "It's a boy, and a girl, and so far they are doing great, and the baby boy looks like my father-in-law." We all laughed it up. My mom cried pretty hard when she heard that one of the babies was a girl. I think she was really hoping for a granddaughter to dress up. My sister's boyfriend smiled and congratulated us. I hugged my husband very tightly, and we decided right there on the names.

About 45 minutes later, my mom's dear friend, who is a NICU nurse, escorted us to the NICU. We were instructed to "scrub in" and put on robes. We did as we were instructed and were welcomed into the NICU. Our son was on a C-pap, which is basically a nasal respirator, and was pretty still. Our daughter was mad. She was fiery and pissy. She had that fightin' spirit that I hoped she would have. Her hair was an awesome pale yellow with wee little ringlets.

We were taught the ins and outs of the NICU and preemies while the bustle of bells and whistles honked and rang around us. We were complimented on the names we had chosen, and told that the babes had the best babysitters in the world taking care of them. A little plug for our NICU, these people are fully responsible for our happiness. Without them, our babies would have died.

Since they were checked into the NICU, the story goes on for 12 more weeks. The biggest issues immediately were who was the legal mother and whose name would go on the birth certificate as the mother. In our state, "the woman who expels the baby" is recognized as the mother. So it was seen that my sister was the mother of these children, for the hospital's records. My sister waived the rights to consent to anything that needed to be performed on the kids, but, while in the hospital, the children's last name was my sister's last name until they were discharged. About two hours after the babes were born, an attorney we had hired to perform a transaction in court so that my name would go on the birth certificate showed up to have all the official paperwork signed. The problem was, when he showed up, my sister had a morphine drip, so she was not seen to have a "sound mind" at the time of signature. That was quite a glitch, since time was of the essence. If we did not get the forms into the court in time, my name would not have been put on the birth certificates for six months or so, and even then, my name would have been added next to my sister's name. None of us wanted that. We wanted my name on my biological children's birth certificates, and my sister wanted to go back to being called "Aunt" legally. Our attorney returned the following day for the signatures. The attorney informed us that the judge on the bench that day was a Catholic, and sometimes they disagreed morally with this particular situation. I guess he was in a good mood that day, because he approved the name switch on the birth certificates, and everything worked out smoothly, for a change.

The story goes on and on. Let's just summarize it this way: 12 weeks in the NICU and five surgeries on the babies' small intestines. We lived in a hotel for 12 weeks and, two jealous dogs later, our babies came home from the hospital, happy and healthy. We were exhausted. It was the best feeling in the world.

It is interesting to look back and remember all of the things that happened to us. I noticed that we have taken so many things for granted. I have to admit that I harbor some jealousy for people who can plan on getting pregnant and have undoubted success. We certainly did not just say to each other, "Let's get pregnant in six months," hop into bed, have sex, and poof, a baby was born 40 weeks later. There are so many stories like that. Yet I do not think the people who have ease getting pregnant have the privileges we had while attempting to have children. To have our babies, as you have just read, we needed a lot of help. In order to get help, we needed to have the support of so many people. Without the help we were given, we would probably have 100 fewer people in our lives, including the first doctor who told me not to get pregnant, the first and second fertility centers, and the wonderful people at the pharmacy where we got all of our IVF drugs, who to this day get so excited when we come in for a prescription refill and give four handfuls of lollipops to the kids. These are people who helped us achieve our dreams, not theirs. This proves to me that there is good in this crazy world. I cannot express the gratitude I have for people in the world who do their work with passion and skill. I cannot thank the people at the fertility center enough for their kindness and understanding and great skill. I cannot thank the people in the hospital and the NICU for their awesome patience with all of the challenges that arose. They seemed to really love not only their jobs but to really love us.

I know you are thinking, "Come on." But I wholeheartedly feel that these people went way above and beyond the expectations of their job description to help our family. Many times people have referred to our kids as "miracles." I have an awful time relying on a higher power to do his or her job and I do not believe in miracles. I do, however, believe in people with passion and skill dedicating their abilities above and beyond what is expected—from an IVF nurse who called us into the office just so she could see the expressions on our faces when she gave us our first good news in three years to the neonatologist who spent four days straight at the NICU just in case anything else happened to our kids. When the neonatologist finally went home to spend time with his family, another surgery had to happen, and he had the surgery dictated to him on his cell phone while he raced back to the hospital, with his very sweet son tagging along.

If these people are here to perform miracles, then I suppose my definition is a little different than most people's definition. If "people with passion" is the definition of miracle, then I guess I do believe in miracles. If the belief that a higher power is in charge is the definition of miracle then I have to resist because I am still angry and I'm okay with that.

Above all, the person I have to thank the most is my sister. For the last three years, I have not found the words to express my feelings. I have written notes and not sent them. I have dialed her number and hung up. I have tried on so many occasions to say "Thanks" but it just isn't enough. My awesome sister took time away from her own life to experience my pregnancy. She is an amazing person, an amazing sister, an amazing friend, an amazing woman and, above all, a totally amazing aunt. I carry a small piece of paper in my wallet that has a quote written on it: "When I count my blessings, I count you twice." I carry that quote so I can always be thankful to her. When I look back at my kids in their car seats, I thank my sister. When I kiss my kids on their heads at bedtime, I thank my sister. When I take a deep breath, and know I have my health, and a happy family, I thank my sister. Without my sister, I would not be the person I am today. For that I am very thankful. The only way I can ever repay her is to raise two incredible people who hopefully will perform miracles someday.

When my sister was 24 weeks pregnant, I made a plaster mold of her round belly. Our plan was to make a mold every month to document the babies' growth. For obvious reasons, we did not get to make a second mold. That mold is on a low shelf in our bedroom. The kids love to rub the belly and say, "Dat's Aunt Suze's belly." It has always made me smile that the kids have such an accepting tone when it comes to their birth story. One day my son said to me, "Mom, when I was a baby, I grew in your belly with Millie." I responded by saying, "No, pal, you grew in Aunt Suze's belly, but you grew in Mommy's heart." He was so accepting of the explanation. Whenever we see a pregnant woman, the kids tell her, "We didn't grow in Mommy's belly, we grew in her heart." The thought is very simple, yet very, very true. My kids are lucky enough to "get" how amazing they really are. Some people never realize how lucky they are, and my two 3-year-olds totally "get it."

As for my childhood fantasy, I obviously never imagined that my pregnancy would have been an out of body experience. I never imagined that I would be so strong that I would overcome life's challenges and go on to try to help other people learn from their life's challenges. I still have dreams that I wake up and I have a big round pregnant belly and I go into labor and my husband is by my bedside while I give birth to our baby. I imagine being so tired and scared and happy all at the same time. I imagine being protective and all knowing. I imagine being glad that everything is okay.

Then I wake up to the sound of one of my kids calling, "Mom, I'm awake and I need muffins and juice!" And I realize that I am living my dream.

2

On the Day Sage was Born

Annalysa Lovos

Some things in life a person just knows. When I first met my future husband, Dave, I knew that I could spend a lifetime with him. I also knew, long before I ever laid eyes on him, that if I were to bear children I wanted to do so at home, in the intimacy of my own bedroom. It seemed only natural to me that the family home must be the most comforting atmosphere to be born into.

But when a head-on collision in my early twenties left me in a wheelchair, many of my activities and beliefs had to be reevaluated, re-created, or set aside. Still, my inner conviction that home was the right place for me to have a baby grew only stronger.

I know you can't always predict these things. Many things can go wrong in childbirth, and in some situations, emergency medical procedures are absolutely necessary. So initially, when Dave and I had pieced together the surprising and wonderful clues that we were pregnant, we talked with many of the doctors, nurses, and specialists I had had occasion to consult with in the past. All of them believed I could have an easy, natural childbirth. And every one of them advised me to do so in the safety of the hospital.

I wanted my birthing experience to be a deliberate, conscious, joyous event—not merely an anesthetized, perfunctory salute to the medical modus operandi. But I also had to accept that, no matter what I wished, it was possible that it might be best for me—and for my baby—to compromise. The relative unknown of paraplegic delivery makes doctors quick to label it high-risk. Even though I didn't feel I was a high-risk patient, I heard their admonitions and dutifully went for a prenatal consultation with the most respected obstetrician I could find.

The first question she asked was, "What medications will you be using?" I was taken aback. Apparently, "No medications" is not a frequent request in labor and delivery these days. It was obvious that a hospital birth was not the experience I wanted. If one expects complications, I thought, then birthing in the hospital is a safe choice. On the other hand, if one is educated about the risks of all-too-common birth interventions and is confident about birthing at home, then the hospital is safest as a backup choice. I didn't expect complications, and I believed—and still believe—in the power one's expectations have to influence outcomes. I also believed in my intuition that homebirth was right for me.

We went home and called a midwife, Marimikel Penn. "Wonderful!" she said. "You can absolutely have a homebirth. Honey, you're going to do great." Marimikel inspired confidence from our very first exchange. She was exactly the woman I wanted to have on my team.

Marimikel is no newcomer to midwifery. When we met her, she had been delivering babies at home—more than 2,000 of them—for 28 years. Only seven percent of her patients have had cesarean sections, while the average for hospital births in the same city of Austin, Texas, is 25 percent. She also gives much more thorough prenatal and postpartum care than a woman is likely to get from an obstetrician, and shares so much supportive knowledge that it would be impossible to go through a birth with her and not feel empowered by the experience.

Dave and I felt great about our decision to work with Marimikel. The hospital was a mere five-minute drive from our home, and she had excellent backup support there if we were to need it. But I was confident that we would not. I believe she was, too—otherwise, she would not have agreed to work with me. Having trained originally as a nurse, Marimikel knew exactly what I meant when I said "paraplegic." She and I shared a strong feeling that things would go well.

Pregnancy was a wonderful time. I felt healthy and enjoyed my growing roundness. I was blessed to have the time to take care of myself the way I wanted and to read everything I could find on homebirth. The hardest parts for me were finding graceful ways to get me and my big belly in and out of my wheelchair—and, of course, having to empty my bladder so frequently.

Three days past my due date, I woke up and prepared for an 8 a.m. appointment with Meredith Kline, the young midwife who would assist Marimikel at our birth. I felt that this could be the day, and so was discouraged when Meredith concluded that I wasn't in labor. Yet not long after she left, contractions began, then stabilized at ten minutes apart. This in itself was nothing new, but I had a slight backache too. I decided to lie down, and Dave called in late to work on a hunch that something was up.

After the contractions, still ten minutes apart, had continued for about an hour, we called the birth center and left a message to alert them, just in case anything came of it. By the time they called back 20 minutes later, the contractions were more intense and only four minutes apart. I was breathing with them. Marimikel said it sounded as if we were going to have our baby today, and that she would be over soon.

Relief and excitement. I was not destined to be pregnant for the rest of my life, after all!

I soon felt that the birth was coming on much faster than we had thought it would. Dave called the birth center and begged them to hurry. On the other end of the line, I heard Marimikel yell to Meredith to drop everything, get the birth supplies in the car, and get to our house. Thankfully, the center was only five minutes from our door. Any farther and they might not have made it in time.

Immediately after they hung up, an enormous rush of energy whooshed through my entire body, curling and shaking me, accompanied by the sensation of a baby rocketing down my birth canal. I don't know through what faculty I felt this, but it was as unmistakable a feeling as the one that tells you you're about to vomit—which I also felt like doing. Something had most certainly moved inside me, and it was awesome and scary to realize that I was not in control of it. I breathed slowly and carefully, and began to hope that if I could hold out for only a few minutes more, the midwives would get there and everything would go smoothly.

On the Day Sage was Born

As for Dave, these were formidable moments. He pushed up his sleeves, found the sheet titled "What to Do in the Event of an Unassisted Birth," and prepared to catch the baby. "I wish Marimikel would get here," he said quietly. These words sank in for a long moment.

Marimikel burst through the door. Without pausing, she jumped onto the bed to size up the situation. "OK, we're gonna have a baby *right now!*" she said. "Annalysa, take a deep breath, and push with the next contraction." The baby's head was beginning to crown.

I had planned to push either on my hands and knees or sitting on a birthing stool, but as it turned out, there was no time to move from the side-lying position I'd been lounging in during early labor.

Marimikel told me exactly how to breathe, and I did my best to follow her directions even through the intense, ripping sensations of labor. I have never felt so much energy in my body as I did then—I now know why pregnant women practice breathing. At the next contraction, Meredith appeared by my side, and, working with Marimikel as if they were two fibers of the same muscle, she applied downward pressure to the fundus of my rock-hard belly with each push, trying to help my half-paralyzed abdominal muscles get the baby out.

It seemed, though, that my body was able to manage the job, for within minutes of Marimikel's arrival, the baby's head and top shoulder emerged. With the next push, the bottom shoulder, then the entire body, shot out into Dave's waiting hands. It felt like a great, pressurized cork had been liberated. Marimikel helped Dave guide the impossibly slick, pink and purple newborn onto my belly, where she cleared its throat. The baby let out a lusty cry and we all shed tears of joy.

Sarah Katherine Sage Lovos weighed seven pounds three ounces and was 19 inches long. She held up her head—wobbly but determined—right away on that first day, and she smiled within an hour of her birth.

We had been right about the birth being an easy one. Maybe my paraplegia actually worked to my advantage, giving my baby an easy passage through pelvic muscles that, in an able-bodied woman, carry much more tension. Maybe it was my expectation of a smooth birth, or maybe simply genetics. The actual labor lasted three hours, and I had been sure of it just in the last 45 minutes. The midwives were bubbling about it; Meredith laughingly called me a Birthing Goddess.

During and right after Sage's birth, I was energetic and happy. But by the time I'd finished chanting her a song of welcome, she had been born for 15 minutes and I looked absolutely peaked. My body had begun to shake, hard and uncontrollably. Rather than nurse her as I'd intended, I was forced to hand Sage off to Dave. The midwives began to look concerned.

My body had sailed smoothly through the birth but I was humbled when it reacted afterward with a high temperature and the shakes. The midwives were quick to jump to my aid; they called the backup doctor and began covering my body with bath towels soaked in ice water. This felt both wonderfully cooling and painfully agitating, which made it even more of a challenge to relax, breathe deeply, and stop the shaking, which was so strong my teeth chattered. I drank several quarts of cold liquid through a straw and thought about how, even though I was dangerously hot, I knew I was OK. I used every scrap of mental power I possessed to calm and cool my bewildered body and assure my attendants that we did not need to go to the hospital.

To everyone's relief, my temperature began to creep down almost immediately. After several changes of towels, my temperature was again normal, but the shaking took longer to pass. Finally, an hour and a half after Sage's birth, I felt normal again and was able to nurse her.

Marimikel, who had been quite worried, stayed for several hours to make sure I was well. Her take on the situation was that it was related to oxytocin, the hormone that causes contractions and induces birth. She thought that my body had released more oxytocin than normal to compensate for the paraplegia, and that it was this energy coursing through me that had caused the heat and shaking. She felt that if I were to have a second baby, my body would be more on target about the right quantity of hormone to produce.

My greatest ally in managing a newborn on my own was the baby sling. Being in a chair and trying to carry a baby at the same time felt not unlike having both arms and both legs tied behind my back. The baby sling, and later a front-pack, freed my arms and let me accomplish things while holding Sage. She loved being carried, and now, at two, still spends plenty of time riding on my lap. We hear daily comments that "She's getting a free ride" or "She's got the best seat in the house."

Having the baby sleep with us for as long as she is nursing has also been a natural solution. Neither Dave nor I is keen on getting up in the middle of the night, and because I park my wheelchair right next to my side of the bed, a cosleeper or crib next to me was not an option. The answer was obvious: get a bigger bed. We also liked the idea that family sleeping helps babies learn their parents' sleeping patterns, which makes the whole family happier and healthier.

Sometimes, as I drift off watching her sleep, I wonder if the path of Sage's life would have been different had she been born in a hospital rather than at home. Sage is bright, energetic, and precocious. Her eyes shine, and it's obvious that nothing slips by her unnoticed. Maybe she would have been the same way had we listened to the doctors and gone to the hospital, but I like to believe that she benefited in many ways from our choice of a natural, comfortable birth in circumstances we knew were right for us.

I think back to Sage's birth with satisfaction, knowing that, somehow, I was guided into making the best choice I could have made for her arrival. The mere fact that I am disabled was, in the end, not a good enough reason to go along with a convention my heart could not justify. My greatest hope is that, with this choice, I have started Sage off on the path of listening to her own inner voice. Whatever path she takes with her own life's journey, I hope she will always take time to value what her most trusted advisor—her heart—tells her.

3

The Mending Cry

Michelle Richards

But rising like an iridescent bubble
Above the suctioning chaos,
A gasp of a life.

The miraculous gasp of a life I have known always
But never touched.
The one that shared my breath until this moment.
The mending cry.

Our New Year began with a bang. On the afternoon of December 31, 1998, we watched from rustled Marriott sheets as the snow swirled past our 23rd floor window and across the street, christening the new Cleveland Browns Stadium. The heartland had never felt more like home....but it wasn't, so after the last piece of confetti drifted slowly to the floor, we returned to Florida. And to our great joy, January ended with no period.

My husband had just turned 48, I was turning 33 in February, and on September 25, 1999, we would have another birthday to celebrate. This baby was the first for each of us, and after much wanting and waiting we were ready, or so we thought.

As educated, more "mature" first timers, my husband and I took all of the classes and read all of the books. We gazed with astonishing wonder at the weekly illustrations and celebrated the new developments of our "grain of rice." The proud daddy-to-be read Dr. Seuss to my expanding tummy and test-drove every stroller he could find. I followed all the rules: no alcohol, limited caffeine, and lots of veggies. Each morning I choked down a prenatal cannon ball, only to taste its reverberations all day, because it was the best thing for our little Emily.

Like the perfect storm, my first trimester of pregnancy collided with my last semester of graduate school, not to mention the long awaited segue into a new career. When I became too seasick to make the 45-minute drive, my studies were surrendered to the greater cause. I had everything mapped out anyway, and when the storm subsided, I told myself, life would resume as usual.

We planned, in writing as recommended, to have a natural birth. The idea of an epidural terrified me, with its endless needle, possible side effects, and besides, being a Romantic at heart, I didn't want to miss a thing. I decided I would spend the first two years at home with our daughter, during which I would breastfeed for a full year while writing my master's thesis on Sylvia Plath. A second child, a boy, would closely follow Emily's smooth transition to pre-preschool.

The "smooth" part wasn't to be. Even in-utero, Emily proved to be fiercely independent. Two hurricanes and one week after her due date, the doctors decided to give her a hand. They had to physically "ripen" my cervix, manually break my water, and chemically induce labor; so much for nature. "Oh, and by the way," the doctor said, "there are traces of meconium in the water, so we'll have a specialist check her as soon as she's out." Looking at what could not have been a pleasant motherly face, he added a quick, "Don't worry, it's routine."

His thundering words began to dissipate at about four centimeters when I began to beg for an epidural. The staff was compassionate and gave me a "relaxing" pill while I waited for the anesthesiologist (after which I casually peed on the floor while further waiting for someone to unhook my many wired appendages). I no longer feared the extended ice pick inching its way into my spine, in fact, at that point I would have let the night custodian administer it. I no longer cared whether I could help push, and as it turned out, I was a lousy pusher anyway. I know, because the epidural wore off at nine centimeters, just in time for a shift change, but a good two hours shy of delivery.

Nurse Ratched took over for Debbie and Jenn and I spent the next hour on one hip trying to turn my floating acrobat. I thought she was getting close when the doctor returned. Maybe it was the drugs, maybe the pain, but I had heard all of the stories about how the one-gloved doctor rushes through the door just as the baby shoots out: "Pop fly, and a spectacular catch!" But not our baby girl, she was "hanging on to my ribs," as her father likes to tell it, and the doctor had to try to pull her out with a suction cup.

On the first attempt, the cup popped off, giving my single, 27-year-old sister a distinct feel for the miracle she was witnessing. But Kim is a smart, resourceful young woman who somehow managed to hold one leg, work the video camera, and still wipe the birth-stew from her face. My wide-eyed husband, who was in charge of the other leg, was grateful for the good doctor's warning that if the cup came off, Emily's head would not come with it.

On the second try, the most miraculous moment of my life happened. It was October 1, 1999, and at 9:17 p.m. I finally heard the words I had waited 41 weeks and over 13 hours to hear: "Stop pushing." All 14 and 1/2 inches of her head made it through the ten centimeters God provided, the additional few the doctor provided, and several more courtesy of moi. The cord was easily removed from around her neck and she slipped out and into two gloved hands. The doctor held her up and I saw Emily Margaret for the first time. She looked rather annoyed. Her dad cut the cord and the medical staff promptly whisked her off for the usual vitals and the "don't worry" examination.

Emily's cry was strong and she was even stronger. Her father's familiar voice lulled her into a hush as she wrapped her dewy new hand around his finger like an exotic bird, even as the doctors poked and measured. We had done something very right. I tried to concentrate on my pride and not on the American quilt my G.Y.N. was surely stitching between my legs. After nearly an hour, I was able to hold my baby for the first time. I was sitting on a bloody diaper of ice, but she was healthy and beautiful and everything was going to be perfect. I did not know the really hard part was just beginning.

At home, I soon realized that the cord cutting had been a grand illusion. Breastfeeding, while warm and cuddly the first dozen hours, became a miserable, never ending stretch of bed rest with the dog, egret-eyed and perched over my bovine side. My heavy breasts were too cumbersome to be a walking milk dispenser, so my "full year" of breastfeeding dwindled to six months, and then anxiously to one.

By the end of the first week I didn't want to get out of bed. I wrote:

Rain gutters drain

Their tin parade.

It's 3 a.m.

I had vaginal stitches and a bladder infection. I ate raisin toast and Tylenol. I cried when Emily cried, I cried when my husband left for work, and I cried again when he returned home, even if he'd only been gone for a couple of hours. Though I was in denial, my melancholy began to show itself:

I ooze, I itch,

No one mentioned

This encore…

I was angry, jealous, and sad. My standard of perfect motherhood was set too high. I held this beautiful child, so thankful, but wondering what I was doing wrong, why it wasn't easier. Motherhood did not feel at all natural. It felt forced, like a smile dragged from an ungrateful guest, like the birth itself. Weeks dawdled into months, so I called the doctor and I took the test. Attached to post-partum depression is the nasty stigma of sensational headlines. But even mild post-partum can enter like a strange and stifling breath that is not so easily exhaled. It brings with it the self-disappointment of a botched rehab:

Distinct etchings vanish

To laboring sameness,

Unrecognizable,

The distortion grows new.

Everything I did felt like failure.

If ever a question deserved thoughtful and honest consideration, "Are you in danger of harming yourself or your child?" is the one. In the eerie stillness of my nurse practitioner's office, I was able to quickly answer "never." Nonetheless the words were sobering, especially when the choices on the standard questionnaire included "sometimes" and "often." Suddenly I was gripped with the realization that it wasn't just me, that with great trepidation, even these other answers were sometimes bubbled in. A calming breath entered my lungs for what felt like the first time, and still I ached for the countless new mothers who were either unwilling or unable to seek professional help. I held each of them in my mind as I wept like an Olympic ice skater waiting for her score.

My renewed heart gradually lightened as I worked hard to recover a recognizable sense of "self." Post-partum depression is kin to post-traumatic stress disorder and the shaken chemicals can be sorted through antidepressants. Because it is a woman's condition, the hormonal imbalance can be stabilized by common oral contraceptives, but the illness is very individual and finding the "right" dosage was basic trial and error. So after four new brands of birth control pills and three different antidepressants, I was finally beginning to glimpse me in the mirror. While regulating the medication, I was also spending many Saturday afternoons bidding farewell to personal demons from a counselor's couch, as well as through my cathartic pen:

> ....today I hate the twig thin
>
> Attorney, mother of three
>
> Tres fashionably poised, polished,
>
> And not even half a Prozac.

Just as children don't come with instructions, neither do post-partum women. At the time, my husband's support was as invisible as the beams of a city skyscraper, but nevertheless what keeps it from crashing down. In retrospect, to no fault of his own, this amazing man was unsure of what to say or when to say it, whether to hold me or to give me space; but he never once faltered as a strong and loving presence for my splintered selves. Make no mistake: parenthood changes you and your life forever. It is an instant marriage, no flirting, no courting, and it takes some getting used to, whether it's part of the plan or not. I had to allow myself ample time, over two years as it turned out, to make all of the necessary adjustments. As I was writing the final chapter of my thesis, I was taking the last doses of my antidepressant and wishing that Sylvia Plath had done the same.

Our lives would be sadly empty without Emily, but we are not brave enough to try for the boy. I am proud, and still quite amazed, at my role in the creation of this olive-eyed little person with a sandy version of her daddy's cowlick. The decision to allow her to be labeled an "only child," like most parental decisions, has inflicted its share of guilt:

> When our shaky twilight
>
> Encroaches your charge,
>
> Cling to those friends, lovers....
>
> There will be no blood link.

I've discovered that motherhood is a dichotomous state of being, but I have also learned that June Cleaver and Mrs. "C" are myths, just like coming out of the delivery room with full make-up and fluffy hair. In essence, I've accepted that Emily Margaret is perfect, and I don't have to be.

4

The Birth Story of Miles

Elisabeth Aron

I remember everything about that morning. I remember thinking, *Remember every moment as it will be the last time that you give birth: the last time you are pregnant, the last time you will be in labor. Remember, so that you can tell him years later the details of how he came into this world.* I remember that I was wearing a black V-neck T shirt and maternity jeans and black Doc Martens. I remember leaving the house before my two-year-old was awake, kissing my husband goodbye, and driving myself to the hospital. I remember thinking about all of the possible things that could go wrong, but by the end I would return with my new addition.

The induction began in a routine fashion. As an OB/GYN myself, I had struggled over whether to try to have a Vaginal Birth After Cesarean (VBAC) or just go for the repeat cesarean section. I decided on trying to deliver vaginally so that I would be better able to take care of my two-year-old and keep her life disruptions to a minimum. I also felt that I should follow the advice I gave to hundreds of patients, that there should be one set of rules for everyone.

Eventually my husband arrived, now that our daughter was fed, dressed, and happily playing at a friend's house. The day was calm and peaceful and we chatted about the future in relative peace. I got my epidural, my doctor broke my water, and things progressed. Ten centimeters dilated arrived right on schedule. I allowed myself to think that this might actually work, that I might actually deliver vaginally. That my decision to try to labor was correct and all was right with the world. My husband even mused that this was much better than last time as he excitedly prepared to start coaching me in the pushing process.

Then all of our lives changed although we didn't even seem to notice while it was happening. The posterior wall of my uterus had ruptured and the baby died inside of the place that had helped it to grow and thrive. In retrospect, all of the signs that something was going wrong were there, but were not clearly seen at the time. Errors in judgment became the groundwork for new errors. The monitor recorded my elevated heart rate while my baby was dying inside of me in front of numerous witnesses. After pushing for an hour, my doctor became concerned about the baby's heart rate and I was rushed back for an emergency cesarean section. As in most emergencies, my husband was forced to wait outside, imagining the worst. I was intubated and so all memory was lost until I awoke in the recovery room.

I remember asking, "Is he all right?" My answer came as my husband bent over to hug me and started crying. The baby had died. Miles was dead.

I wanted to see him and as soon as the anesthesia had worn off enough and I could keep my eyes open, they gave him to me. He was dressed in a ridiculous outfit that must have been collected and saved for situations like these. I undressed him and looked at all of his body parts individually. He was so beautiful and new and perfect. Then I placed his naked body against mine and just held him while tears poured from my heart. The thing that I remember most is how he smelled. Someone, someone who I never met or got to thank, had washed him, had made him smell deliciously clean, and then had lovingly dressed him. Someone had understood that this is what I would remember and that he was important enough to have gone through this newborn ritual. Someone had taken care of him, as I would have, while I was unconscious in the operating room. That same someone had also lovingly taken pictures of him in various poses, dressed and undressed, to document his existence. Although I do not wish to meet that person, she must know that doing these things meant more to me than words could ever express.

I needed to hold Miles again the following day. Even though not all of my family agreed to see him, I needed to show him to my family to prove that he had been here. My sister-in-law picked up the corpse, dressed and swaddled, held him close, and announced to the world, "I love you and I will always love you." When I remember that day, it is this moment that that brings me the most tears: there are loving, open people in this world who feel deeply.

It's been several years since the birth and death of our baby. He still lives among us, but life has gone on. I am thankful that this was not my first child. My daughter forced me to go on with the day-to-day needs of life. Her smiles and laughter have made us recover faster. The most difficult thing for me now is to look at pregnant women, which has made my profession a little harder to work in. I know in my head that most, if not all, will be bringing home babies. But I worry that they will not, that they could experience the same loss that I have. They are so full of hope.

We are expecting again. This time it is a child from Korea. He will magically arrive on an airplane without epidurals, IVs, or surgery. It will be a painless delivery, for me. As I look at pregnant women and see the possibility of future sorrow, I also look at the arrival of our new child as a great source of sorrow for his mother.

How do you give up a child? How do you recover from that pain? I guess you just go on and a small part of you never gives him up. I still look at his picture everyday. I still think about my birth story every time I do a delivery. He is still with me.

If memories keep your hopes and dreams alive, I hope that my son's mother will have some good memories to get her through the difficult days that lie ahead. A picture, a footprint, a loving glance. My wish is that his mother knows that he is safe and clean and loved. In honor of his mother, I will try to remember every minute of the day of his arrival into our lives, so that I can tell him how he came to live with us and be ours.

5

Largesse

Jennifer Mattern

lar•gesse n. [Old French < LARGE] 1. generous giving, as from a patron 2. a gift or gifts given in a generous, or sometimes showy, way 3. nobility of spirit

I overshot the runway.

There is no going back, no possibility for graceful retreat. I ate too much, too soon. This is what I am told. I am told many things, every day, now, by my doctor, family, friends, strangers. *I am told. I am instructed. I am scheduled. I am tested.* During my pregnancy, the passive voice is omnipresent and inescapable. *I am submerged.*

The active voice had been my dominion, equal parts turf and prerogative. *Veni, vidi, vici*—more *veni* and *vidi* than *vici*, perhaps, but I held my own. Now, I am with child, and I must receive before I may deliver. It is unfamiliar terrain, a meek new world. Here, I am the recipient of copious advice, mostly unsolicited. It is administered to me daily by the natives, pressed damply into my palms, ears, *you'll need this.* I am the recipient of touch, the touch of strangers. They lay hands on me in subway cars, in public restrooms, eager to heal what is not broken. I do not speak their language, so instead I smile, helplessly. Their customs are strange, but for the most part, they are kind, even as they pass comment on my largeness, *big as a house, already.*

I am as big as a house; I am the house I am building. *Mi casa, su casa.* I would tell them this if I could: I am a construction worker, laying rows of *penne rigati* as foundation for the unborn, cementing take-out cartons of *aloo gobi* as cornerstones, smoothing enchilada bricks into place with sour cream. I am a skilled laborer; expansion comes easy to me. I wink at tittering old women as they pass me on the sidewalk. *Morning, ma'am. Please step back, ladies, building a baby, here.* Evidence of my construction appears on my spreading ass, on my chafing thighs. The cellulite is conspicuous, sloppily spread mortar.

Eat, eat, this city croons to me, morning till night. The melting pot has spoken, and I dip my ladle into it again and again, grateful for the invitation to partake. I am eating for two, four, eight, the world. Thai. Ethiopian. Russian. I imagine my unborn child floating in a sea of rich, oily chicken broth, *pelmeni* dumplings dancing about her head, a wreath of doughy crescent moons adorning a smiling, belching cherub.

I have always been a sturdy woman, a woman of enthusiastic appetites, but this eating is deadly serious business. I now hunger with a shocking urgency. I hunger with violence. I must have what I must have. "You have to cut back," my doctor warns, frowning and clicking her pen, *in-out-in-out.* "Your weight gain is more than ideal." My doctor is also pregnant, but diminutively so. Her pregnancy has the take-it-or-leave-it aesthetic of the hasty addition of a purse or a belt or a shawl. An accessory, easily shed, *what, this old thing?*

I have nothing to shed. I am the pregnancy; I have been consumed by it. My former frame has been folded into a thick batter that continues to rise, spilling out of its loaf pan in fat white dollops. Each morning, I regard my burgeoning reflection, and I am humbled by my own bounty. The mirror does not lie. I am manna from heaven, I am raining loaves and fishes. I know what I am seeing—there is grace at work, here.

But I am large, I concern multitudes. My mother, especially, is concerned. My mother is concerned that I am not concerned. She and my doctor do not see the loaves, the fishes. "You still have a long way to go, remember," she points out. "I'm listening to my body," I tell her. "It wants what it wants." A long pause, then she replies, "Maybe it's time for a little self-restraint."

Largesse

My doctor orders more tests—*I am tested*—to make sure all is well, in spite of my size. She begins her maternity leave tomorrow, and she is brusque. "If this baby gets any bigger," she says grimly, "you'll be on the fast track to a c-section." I am quietly pleased. I, who cannot keep a plant alive for more than three months—a trimester—am growing within me a gigantic hothouse tomato of a baby. I will take first prize at the county fair. People will come from far and wide to have their pictures snapped beside my enormous offspring. Hundreds will line up to play "Guess the Baby's Weight," and before the night is through, one lucky winner will take home a gift certificate to the local steakhouse. My doctor will make a special appearance with her thin, unsmiling family to present me with the key to her suburb. *I knew she had it in her,* she will say, primly. The crowd will cheer as I nurse my infant in our pen, the one usually reserved for the prize hogs.

My mother does not want to hear about the county fair. "You need to listen to your doctor," she says. "Your brother was almost ten pounds. He ripped me wide open." I cannot imagine the child inside me ripping me open, tearing me asunder. Not this child. She is too gentle, too liquid, in her movements. She stretches, does not strike. She squirms, never kicks. I defend her silently to my jury of one, before there is any crime committed.

"What does David say about your weight gain?" my mother demands. "Put him on the phone." "He's not worried about my weight," I tell her. "He's worried about our spoons." David, my husband, believes that I have inadvertently disposed of all but three of our teaspoons. His theory: I absentmindedly left them to drown in the milky bottoms of empty half-gallon ice-cream cartons, which I later discarded. It is a sound theory, one that he is reluctant to impart. He is not angry about the loss of the spoons; he is only concerned that the pattern may have been discontinued. It is a simple, elegant pattern named *Audrey* or *Chloe* or *Paige* (we cannot remember which, and this will be our ultimate flatware-matching doom). Audrey (for the sake of argument) sports an attractive flared handle with a ridge down the center. It reminds me of the dark line on my belly that has appeared within the past few months, snaking its way below my waistband: *linea nigra*, the pregnancy books call it. The black line. *The teaspoons took the four o'clock Linea Nigra to Terra Incognita.*

I wonder what is happening in the terra incognita within my bulk, why I am not feeling more movement. "Sometimes it's difficult for a larger woman to feel the baby moving," Gatekeeper Nurse sighs, over the phone. I call the doctor's office only rarely, but Gatekeeper Nurse is irritated nonetheless. She fields tens of calls each day from anxious mothers-to-be, *is that normal? and this?* I am one of their many beggars, all seeking more than they have to offer, or are willing to give. Gatekeeper Nurse hangs up before I can add—*just one more thing*—that this baby is in no hurry to make her way to the starting gate—*a problem?* We are coming down to the wire, and my child is still stretched horizontally in my womb, an inner equator. "She's still lying sideways," I tell my husband, who never doubts that grace is on our side. "For all we know, she'll crawl sideways through life," I say. He considers this, teaspoons temporarily forgotten. "Well," he says gently, "we want her to be special."

At the baby shower, my mother's Polish cousins ply me with boiled *kielbasa* and sauerkraut, homemade lasagna, potato salad. "Don't you worry about the weight," says one. "You're helping God make a miracle." "You look *wonderful*," gushes another. "Pregnancy agrees with you," says a third. The white cake, decorated with pink sugar roses, bears an inscription to my daughter, in blue icing: *We Love You Already.* My nephew, now a young man, taps insistently on my shoulder. He shows me his beloved Special Olympics gold medal, presented to him by his hero, Arnold Schwarzenegger. "Jenn," he says, shaking his head in disbelief, "you're so *big*." He grins and flings his lanky arms around me, refusing to let go. I hug him back, marveling at his surprising strength. I wonder where he has been hiding it, why I have not noticed it before.

My husband and I bring home two carloads of gifts. *I am showered.* Crocheted blankets, crib sheets, a car seat, stuffed lambs and bears, stacking cups, lacy dresses, diaper bags, diaper cream, and bottles of baby bath cram the foyer of our small apartment. There is no crib, not yet. I wonder how it will fit through the door. "They pack them flat," my husband explains. I think of my grandmother, long dead. When my mother was pregnant with me, my grandmother kindly assured her that labor pains were a myth, saying, of babies, "They expand when they hit the air."

44

Largesse

Time slows. My pace slows. I lumber, I shuffle, a benevolent, foraging bear in the big city, cradling my belly in my arms. In front of our apartment building, trying to get a better look at the dumpster on fire in the schoolyard across the way—*damn kids, third time this week*—I lose my balance and lurch, flailing from the curb into the street, a vertical drop of eight inches. An audible *pop*: my left ankle buckles beneath my weight. The pain is astounding. Wedged between the bumpers of two black SUVs, unable to speak or stand, I claw frantically at the air. Passersby do just that, scrutinizing bricks, sidewalk cracks, rubbish in the act of passing—anything but the large, whimpering woman in the gutter. I notice a pair of dark-eyed children watching me with great interest from behind the bars of their first-floor apartment window. Still mute with pain, I beckon to them. Alarmed, they yank the curtains closed.

A wraith of a man appears on the curb beside me. "I fell, I'm pregnant," I whisper, as if this is simple cause-and-effect at work, as if the fall is to blame for my gravid state. *I am fallen.* He struggles to free me from the vise of the SUVs, but my ankle is wedged in the sewer grate, and my mass is no match for him. After several unsuccessful attempts to pull me to my good foot, he encourages me to use one of the SUVs for leverage. With his assistance, I scale the hood of the larger vehicle. The dumpster is still burning. A small crowd has gathered across the street to watch and cluck. *Kids. Unbelievable.*

I can bear no weight on my left ankle. My bantam-weight Samaritan timidly takes my arm and lays it across his shoulders. "It's okay," he says, simply. I see now that I am a foot taller than he, and at least 80 pounds heavier. With my human crutch tucked neatly into my armpit, I hobble into the lobby of my building. He is willing to take me further, to my door, to my bed. I wonder suddenly if he knows the savagely unfunny joke: *So the ant says to the elephant, I'll take the thorn out of your foot, if you let me f--- you afterwards.* I quickly dismiss my petite savior from the lobby and make sure he is gone before crawling to the elevator.

The ankle is grotesquely swollen, but it does not look out of place. There is little to be done as it heals. Obediently, I elevate it and ice it hourly. I sleep, I grow, I wait, I eat. Always, I eat. Emancipated from my daily commute and my weekly Metrocard, I am serene. I send my husband off to work. I receive the occasional visitor and hold court when it is required, but for the most part, everything is still. Very little is expected of me. For this, I find that I am deeply, profoundly grateful. I realize that I am tired. I wave my world and my weight ahead of me: *you go on, I'll catch up.*

When I reach 200 pounds, my doctor decides that enough is enough. They will take matters into their own hands and smoke her out, nearly four weeks early. It is for my own good, they tell me. I must, they insist, trust them.

I do not want to release her. My husband watches helplessly as my body clamps down, denying passage for 22 hours. "Don't move so much," a nurse scolds. I do not know these nurses. I cannot tell them apart. "Keep your hands down," the attending physician, another stranger, warns me. "We need a sterile field." I do as I am told. I lie still, determined to be an exquisite field of sterility, the finest they have ever seen. A rolling, overgrazed pasture, cropped clean and bare and colorless by hungry bovines and sheep.

"Do you want a mirror?" one nurse asks. "To help you push?" Before I can respond, she aims a plastic hand mirror directly between my spread legs. The mirror does not lie, and one look tells me all I need to know: *this* is not happening *there. That* is not the bull's-eye they believe it to be. The nurse smiles down at me as I stare at my exposed crotch. She adjusts the mirror helpfully, a hairdresser, *really brings out your eyes.* She expects a modicum of praise for her efforts, I can tell. I can give her this; throughout my labor, I remain inordinately polite. "No, thank you," I say. The nurse seems dismayed by my refusal—miffed, quite possibly—but she acquiesces and removes the mirror. I close my eyes to look for what she cannot offer, for the thing that no one else can see.

When my daughter finally, blessedly, emerges from her place near the center of my enormity, a hush falls over the delivery room. "You've got yourself a little peanut baby," says someone, brightly. "Four pounds!" It is a gruesome tabloid mistake: Switched At Birth. Four pounds is a twin, a triplet, a crack baby, a bag of kibble, a purse. Where is my lush hothouse child? Where is my prize pumpkin? Who has taken her from me? And the parallel tragedy: Whose child is this?

She is beside me, suddenly, wrapped in a candy-striped blanket. Someone—not I—reaches into my hospital gown and exposes my left breast. Anonymous hands push the swaddled infant insistently against my breast and into my arms. I submit, and then, I accept. We squint at each other, she and I, both bleary-eyed and shaken. Concerned strangers, paths crossing for the first time, courtesy of a car accident—no one's fault, just bad weather, a skid of circumstance. *Are you okay? Yes, thank God, you?* "Stay still," the doctor commands. "You tore pretty badly." I look at the small, blinking cornucopia on my chest. *You are bigger than you realize,* I want to say, but she is gone before I can tell her this, whisked away for further examination because of her size. *She is whisked. She is taken. She is examined.* I notice her empty hospital identification band, nestled beside me in the sheets.

It is not until we get home that the passive voice recedes and we finally surface, gasping for air and for each other. *I hold you. I see you.* I stand naked before the full-length mirror to bear witness to us, together, for the first time. My tiny daughter peers quizzically from her perch on my shoulder—the lady of the manor, groggy from a stolen afternoon nap, leaning out the window to see if it will rain. She looks very much at home, needing nothing, wanting nothing, offering nothing but this. *She is. We are.*

My hunger is waning. I search the mirror for evidence that I have diminished in size, but there is none. With my daughter pressed against my bare skin, I am larger than life. Together, we are larger than life. The mirror, I think, does not lie, and I welcome its version of the truth.

6

Untwinning

William Pierce

Naïve man: I thought the births of my two children would hold against time and age, that those hours would preserve their immediacy. They would burrow into some unchangeable redoubt in my mind and become an eternal just-gone-by. The two labored walks to the hospital, the two arrivals of our obstetrician, the two delivery rooms two doors from each other in the same wing and same corridor, would never merge. One time a girl. Once a boy. Each would occupy a distinct pocket of memory—even the word *memory* felt like sacrilege. Each was my unshakable Now. As we left for the hospital again, here they were: our daughter at a neighbor's house, all of my experience of childbirth still at that moment inhering in her (though already: how small had she been, exactly?), and before us, clenched and kicking, a radical uniqueness, his gender not yet known: our son.

A beautiful vision, I'll give myself that. But the mind doesn't work that way. With our son's seventh birthday just gone by, the knot of memory needs a slow teasing-out to give me those two nights distinct. If both events mingle wherever it is that we remember joy, they stretch toward different quadrants—the one ending in first-time wonder, the other in what felt like crisis superhumanly averted.

My wife, Gillian, and I met 22 years ago, in our junior year of college. We were quickly addicted. I admired her wide-ranging intelligence, which was of a different, more fluently recombinatory and inclusive kind than any I'd ever known. And we relied on each other's different kinds of confidence, mine brasher though

48

more limited, hers more firmly intellectual and patinaed with self-doubt. Gillian played classical piano and listened to Elvis Costello and the Smiths; I, the boorish one, slept through her recitals (hung over, though my excuse makes it worse) and listened to AC/DC and the Cars. We both needed books to function.

Flash forward past graduate school and marriage. On July 16, 1998—the day we became parents—we arrived at the hospital too late, which turned out to be just in time. The nurses signed us in, administered doses of matronly Ohio small talk, and then glanced inside. *Your water did break—when did it happen?* Contractions, we knew, had started at the Olive Garden the night before. A pitocin drip was scheduled for two days later—to artificially induce labor—and all through dinner and on the drive home we had congratulated each other for dodging an intervention we didn't want. *You should have come to the hospital last night! Weren't you warned about infection?* Warned, yes, but only now did we realize that the amniotic sac had torn, must have, before I fell asleep. Not wanting to spend an extra minute in the hospital, Gillian had promised to wake me when the right time came, and then paced the house to withstand the contractions, occasionally pausing to snuggle with our dog on the sofa. We were too inexperienced to know—it was a slow leak rather than a gush because our daughter's head was tight against the cervix, an extraordinarily hairy plug. *'Contractions spaced thus-and-so—or whenever your water breaks'!* they chastised, quoting the mantra. But we were secretly pleased: we had walked to the hospital between 7:00 and 7:30, and our daughter joined us at 1:45. It was a wildly short first-time run, and within two hours we were eating pizza in our hospital room.

Revelation, that first time, came with our befuddled stare not at a baby, as we'd expected, but at Catharine, our daughter, whose name seemed as obvious at that moment as her difference from every person yet born—not superiority, we were too new to parenting to have reached that point, but endearing obvious difference.

By the second time, naturally, we were pros, and there were no wrenching decisions to make. Gillian had chosen an epidural before, but under the shocked duress of contractions; this time, without qualm, she would choose one again. The nurses attending Catharine's birth seemed to expect it. *Why be a hero,* their questions implied. *For sure don't avoid it just because your husband expects you to.* And Gillian—rightly, I think now, though the momentarily loosening of our bond confused me—turned toward them, not so much as nurses, but as women; she became of them and released herself to their judgment. To me, as befuddled coach, it was an about-face: under the influence of the usual propaganda, we'd decided—or had I alone decided?—that anesthesia might deprive her of an elemental experience of childbirth and leave her feeling less like a mother. Now almost three years had passed, and we both knew better. The contractions were coming fast and hard, it was late at night, her water had not broken—for sure not broken—and it was time to walk the two blocks to the hospital.

I remember the nurses' quiet surprise. Gillian's cervix was dilated enough for them to call the anesthesiologist. Everything seemed to be moving quickly. But her water hadn't broken.

It was bemused surprise, though. They were trained to expect the usual. And what they saw was a second-time mother. The cervix would dilate further, the sac break, they'd call her obstetrician just in time, and he—like me, I'm reminded— would get as much of his beloved night's sleep as possible. There was no need to call him now, they insisted. And when the cervix did not dilate further, when Gillian's water did not break, never mind. She was a second-time mother. It would all happen fast. In the middle of the night, the anesthesiologist arrived with his kit.

But before the epidural, an I.V.—a peripheral catheter inserted by one of the nurses. The slightest medical invention transforms you from a civilian into a patient, and here we were with the incompetent night shift. Mary or Janine or Pat inserted the needle and missed. She stuck and restuck, a patient plunger, until blood came up the line, finally, a vein releasing its treasure. She thumbed the wheel to pull down drips of saline and reverse the flow. But she was tired, or maybe she worked as a cashier at Wal-Mart and had only come in to play make-believe, who knows. But she didn't secure the needle, and it swung and probed beneath Gillian's skin—my exclamations did nothing to help—until a blister or a veritable pouch of blood gathered beneath the skin of her forearm. Remove needle, begin with step one above. Too shallow, too deep, too shallow, too deep; then, at last, with a wad of cotton and a strip of tan bandage the nurse covered the ingress of her successful pipeline—and no doubt put a red tag on our door, warning others that the husband in Delivery Three was as male as they'd all suspected.

The anesthesiologist, who'd either just now arrived or, I forget, gone to gossip with the nurses or buy something from a vending machine, returned to count Gillian's lowest vertebrae, swab her back with alcohol, and sink a line into her back. I'd lost confidence in everyone around us, but said nothing, and he made no mistakes. Gillian shivered—I knew the weak falling sensation of those spinal and post-spinal manipulations—then rested back as the feeling left her legs. After a time, the anesthesiologist reached under the bed sheet and wiped an alcohol pad across her skin. *Do you feel anything?* She felt it a little. *Does it feel cold?* It felt cool. He talked to her nicely some more. They agreed on a light dose that would let her push so she could feel the birth of her baby. *What about that?* he asked. She felt it, but it wasn't cold. Then, right on schedule, another contraction. It felt like a contraction, she said, but without the pain. The anesthesiologist undid his equipment, packed his bag, and he was gone. At least that's how I remember it. He left the line in her back, just in case, and told the nurses to call with any problems.

Contractions came and went. I stood by Gillian for a while, checked her arm. Then I read. I'd expected to be coaching; a second birth would be quick and intense, we'd thought. But Gillian was tired, and when the epidural took away her pain—and that terrible anticipation of the next hard clenching—she fell asleep. You'll have to excuse the book; it was something ridiculous, an otherwise plausible volume that had no business being in a delivery room. The image in my mind—uncomfortable brown vinyl chair, legs tucked under me, staggered horizontal creases in the beige wallpaper—insists it was Thorstein Veblen's *The Theory of the Leisure Class*.

But I realize now that I'm thinking of Catharine's birth, because when it was Liam's turn, the epidural only seemed to take. Within several contractions it wore off, and Gillian couldn't sleep at all. Her cervix was slightly effaced, but still not opening—four cm, four cm, the baby at negative two station. Any minute now, they were sure, her water would break. *Or it should.* Which meant everything was proceeding as expected. No need for the doctor.

Despite the nurses' confidence, I couldn't read. I'd brought a book with me, I'm sure—probably no less random a book than three years earlier. But whenever the nurses came in, I was standing, ready to query them. When they didn't come, I was in the hall. A long time with no progress, I said, can't we ask the doctor's advice? *We're not calling the doctor. He's asleep. It's the middle of the night. Your wife hasn't reached the required dilation. Her water hasn't broken. We're not calling. It is not time to call. Would you like a juice or a can of soda? Shouldn't you be watching World Wrestling Federation or buffing your car or hitting on the babysitter?*

I tried not to piss them off. We were relying on these nurses for the health, even the life, of our second child. But I pressed, and at 6 or 6:30 in the morning, telepathically successful, my angst must have succeeded in waking the obstetrician in his bed, where he sat up, looked at the clock radio, checked his phone to be sure he could get a dial tone, then humphed and called the hospital to see why they hadn't called about Gillian Pierce. Her contractions were staccato by then, fierce, painful. But no water, no fifth centimeter, and already she was gazing at me with a crooked smile, shrugging, saying at least she was feeling childbirth without the drugs. She looked exhausted—*A Farewell to Arms* exhausted. The resemblance unnerved me.

In the years since then, the elective cesarean has grown from an oddity for the self-pampering few to a distortion for the self-pampering many. Of course, the *non*-elective c-section goes on saving mothers and babies. But for Gillian, surgery for any reason marked a Rubicon, and she didn't want to cross it.

I, on the other hand, had gone to the knife five times already. My father jokes that each medical specialty finds just cause in advising its own services, and as a heart surgeon he raised me in the knowledge that all problems have their corresponding cuts. Two hernia repairs (elective), an ACL reconstruction (elective—I stayed awake to watch), the removal of a lipoma (not even advised by the doctor who did it—he shrugged and opened me in a clinic room with a gaggle of medical students onlooking), and the elision of a mole on my face (not elective: my father abhors beauty marks). Surgery felt routine. But no matter: as the nurses began whispering *cesarean section*, I was full of regrets and fear and helpless anger. What had started with incompetent trowel-work in Gillian's arm had outgrown the nurses' refusal to wake up our doctor and was leading into a mire of technology—procedures making up for procedures making up for procedures— all of it drawing us away from anything our forebears (Caesar notwithstanding) would have recognized as childbirth.

When our obstetrician arrived, smoothly affirming my worst fears by hissing at the nurses—yes, for not waking him up—I began to understand that this was how things happened, how babies were unexpectedly lost, how in the rarest cases a healthy baby began to struggle and finally suffocated, and that anything could happen now: that this was life and death. *What in God's name were you thinking,* the doctor seemed to be hissing at them, and the daytime nurses, the professionally trained ones, just arriving, turned on the lights in the operating room, a visible reproach. *The baby's heart rate isn't up any more than I'd expect after so many hours of hard labor, but we can't let this stress go on much longer—for your wife either,* he told me. Even thinking about it now, pulse quickens. His words weren't dire. Nor was the tone he used in speaking them. But his body smoked with a kind of peeved agitation that told me things weren't going as they should—or rather hadn't gone as they should have.

It will take time to prep the room, but we can have it ready in 20 minutes. He reached between Gillian's legs with a small, sharp, plastic hook and, pushing the baby's head away, snagged the placenta.

Maybe it was then, at that moment of no return, that I started talking to our baby soundlessly. I had nothing else to do. The words were a kind of prayer, but a motivational prayer chanted by a tough coach. Words that seem ridiculous on cold reflection. *Fight through it. Come on.* I was worried about brain damage, of course. Maybe irrationally. New-fatherly. Ersatz-new-motherly too: Gillian was sweating and half asleep, if nowhere near resting. Intermittently she would hyperventilate instead of taking the nice deep breaths we had practiced. Then the contraction would pass again. How many hours of earthquake had there been: seven, eight? And she'd nod to no one, to herself, and give a big puffing sigh. *Come on, get the hell out of there,* I prayed, *wriggle out,* pacing and holding her hand—it was the two-step pace of someone caged, the too-tight hold of a man whose failure to insist, whose failure to *push*, had let go a tumble of consequences that were now endangering his wife.

Scenarios play. Like other imaginations, mine can throw up alternate histories or improbable futures so strongly that the present drops off and another fully propped, palpable world beckons like Marley's ghost. Even in the presence of our fresh-faced doctor, my confidence was gone—I wasn't at all sure that a Caesarian would go well, and didn't want Gillian wheeled across the hall. What were our alternatives? It was my greatest, most frustrating nightmare: to be forced into choosing something bad because the quick spill of fate had left bad and worse.

Somewhere, I returned home by myself. *A Farewell to Arms*, but with a three-year-old to raise. Somewhere else, I lost only one of them, not the other; our second child arrived still-born, and I blamed myself. Elsewhere, we reconfigured our lives to raise a child whose brain the twin snakes of provincialism and stubbornness had deprived of oxygen. All of this while I stood quietly by Gillian's head, watching, stroking, not wanting her to see this unaccustomed fear.

But she, too, had heard the whispers of a Caesarean, and as soon as the obstetrician broke her water, her face changed. She no longer gazed around the room or rested back with her half smile. She crushed my fingers in her hand, but otherwise kept her focus elsewhere.

Afterward she told me that because of that first epidural, the one that had *taken* nearly three years earlier, she had only just now, this second time, learned what nurses and prenatal instructors meant by *pushing*. She hadn't known that it meant push right there, bear down, like that—she hadn't pictured or felt it properly at all. That they meant *push* like a hand inside of you, a new-found hand inside of a woman gently but firmly and insistently pushing the baby out, saying *It's time now, you're coming whether you like or not. You're coming now.*

She stopped looking at me altogether. She stopped looking at the doctor, at the nurses. She looked only up and ahead, locked on to a flower where the wallpaper met the ceiling, and pushed. She pushed madly, with nothing left. But no, not madly: evenly, decisively, single-mindedly. The head, an arm. Take your knives and go to hell.

Untwinning

In those ten minutes, Gillian saved us.

I remember the surprised cries of the doctor. He and the nurses tried to reconfigure the bed for delivery, but they couldn't do it in time. Midway, they gave up, and the OB reached forward and caught our baby in his hands. Our boy. Our son with testicles so large, as I'd never been told to expect, that he seemed to be flashing a neon sign at us: I'm a boy, I'm a boy!

I almost wrote that those first moments diverted me from my hours of anxiety. But they didn't. Gillian had been too tired, too absorbed, for anxiety or fear—and her body's quick forgetting of even that last sharp pain left her deeply available to our son's nuzzlings. But I was the man in the room, the husband and father, a stranger even to myself, and over the next 24 hours, or maybe more, I needed to reconnect, to bring myself back to the innocence I'd felt when we left for the hospital, tote bag in hand. I'd imagined away the simplicity. I'd changed my footing. But here again, Gillian was ready—her mother coming in now, our daughter joining us. Gillian released herself to the instincts of mothering, and again we were saved.

7

Waiting

Ann Angel

My daughter Emily sits in her father's recliner, growing more round each day, more full each hour, more rotund each moment until she appears like a piece of overripe fruit. She's ready to split. She sits in that recliner with eyes closed, rubbing her heavy stretch-marked belly day after day after day. Waiting.

Emily, who should be in school, but is now too big to fit into the desks, too slow to keep up in the halls, and too tired to care, sits in that recliner and sings along with the stereo as it croons love songs and lullabies.

I watch my daughter and know she is nesting. Emily, my firstborn, too young to be a mother herself, moves so slowly now, burdened with the weight of this baby. I watch from the kitchen and see my daughter with skin that glows, her hair pulled back in a French braid. A woman too soon.

She rubs vitamin E and olive oil in circles over the surface that her growing baby has scarred. Her belly has stretched so large that her hands can no longer find the far reaches of skin. She asks me to help her rub the oil in. It is the only small thing I can do to soothe my daughter and her baby.

I squeeze open a capsule of vitamin E and warm the olive oil in my hands before letting it drizzle above my daughter's mammoth womb, and the tender voice from the stereo appeases me.

I use gentle fingers to make small circles over Emily's stomach, rubbing olive oil into red lines that extend like feathers on her white skin. The scars, a momento of the daughter my daughter will hardly know.

Waiting

As I rub, I search for the cushioned shapes that delineate the different parts of this baby, who should have been born weeks ago. I find the solid circumference of her head. I can make out a foot that kicks into skin and muscle. The baby—Emily has already named her Grace—is too large and long to swim now. But she stubbornly refuses to be born. This is her tiny sedition. I can't help thinking she wants to stay, as long as possible, inside this cocoon of mother.

As my hands slip and slide along Emily's skin, soothing the stretch marks, I pray they comfort my daughter's sore heart and sad soul. Baby Grace stirs and shifts as she always does during this ritual of olive oil and E. The head and foot recede beneath my hands and Grace's rump makes itself felt beneath the surface of Emily's skin. I cup my hand around the tiny butt, recalling how much Emily and her siblings loved it when I rubbed and patted them as infants. I tell Emily how I used to rock her to sleep, my hand always circling. Circling her head, her back, her butt. "This baby will be just like you," I tell Emily. I warm more olive oil and drizzle it over the mound of baby. Then I joke, "She's also going to be the queen of olive oil."

It's a stupid joke, really. No better than when Emily comments, now that the baby has taken on so much weight, that walking has become an Olympic feat. But Emily and I, in these final days, make bad jokes in order to ease fear and grief. This is the closest we three generations of women will be in our kinship. Emily's baby, conceived in a loving but too fragile relationship, is another couple's miracle.

I look at the calendar and see that Valentine's Day is only a few days away. This baby should have been born two weeks ago. I tell Emily that her baby must be born soon. And so we walk the mall. We amble past shop windows filled with red ribbons and lacy hearts in preparation for the day of love. We plod past coffee kiosks and candy stores. We walk until Emily can't anymore.

Sometimes we stop because Emily is just too tired. Sometimes Braxton Hicks cramps falsely warn us that now may be the time. But the contractions disappear as soon as we get back home, and Emily settles her great bulk into the recliner. Baby Grace refuses to be born.

Another day goes by. My friend Anita reminds me that it took spicy food to make her kids want to be born, and so I encourage Grace's presence with spicy sausage pizza one day, enchiladas the next. I only give Emily heartburn.

A friend advises that Emily walk again. That will make the baby come. But our Wisconsin weather is unpredictable, frigidly cold one day, drifting snow the next. Emily won't step foot outside because she can't see her feet beneath this mound of baby. She can't stand the mall again; Valentine's in store windows are a sad reminder of love lost and the prices paid.

Besides, Emily says she is too tired, too worn out by the weight of this pregnancy to take another step. So we spend these last few days, Emily in the recliner, rubbing olive oil and vitamin E into stretched and tired skin, singing to baby Grace. *Lullaby and good night, you're your mother's delight. Shining angels beside, my darling abide.*

It is the day before Valentine's Day. The roads are slippery and dangerous with snow, and Emily and I are the only ones at home when her water finally breaks. I call the doctor. I call her father to pick our sons up from their sports practices, and I call the neighbor to send daughter Jeannie home. Emily has asked her little sister to be her birth coach along with me.

I help Emily clean up and settle her into the car next to her sister. We slip and slide all the way to the hospital. It is nine o'clock at night on the 13th of February. We ride in silence. I turn the heat on full blast and pray we make it in one piece. I pray my daughter will be safe. And I pray the baby comes fast. I don't want this baby born on Valentine's Day.

But she is.

Grace, after all her reluctance to come into this world, comes fast, but not fast enough. She is born after only four hours of labor, just a few minutes after midnight on this snowy winter night.

She rests on Emily's already diminishing abdomen, a healthy and beautiful baby girl. When she cries, I rub her rump gently to soothe her. She calms instantly and dozes on Emily. The nurse is amazed that this baby seems to know the feel of my hand against her skin. Emily cradles her little baby girl while her sister Jeannie looks on. When Emily croons lullabies, we swear that Grace recognizes the melody of her voice. We women sit in that night-lit room and watch snow fall out the window, listening to Emily sing. *Sleepyhead, close your eyes. Mother's right here beside you.*

Waiting

We count Grace's perfect fingers and toes and marvel at the way her mouth forms a tiny heart shape. Soon enough, Grace will become someone else's baby girl. For now, she is my daughter's baby; she is Jeannie's first niece, my lovely Valentine granddaughter.

This isn't really my story to tell, it's Emily's. But I tell it anyway because I was so fortunate to have a small part in my daughter's moments with her daughter. It isn't a cautionary tale so much as a story of love and loss. A story of savoring the details of a baby's birth, and of missing the minutiae of that baby growing up.

For three weeks, Emily has the chance to love her baby fiercely, to cradle her in her arms, to sustain her with food and song. Our family takes turns passing baby Grace from arm into arm, loving her completely. We marvel at each little movement, the sweet sounds that whisper and coo through those infant lips. Jeannie is sure the baby smiles just for her. My husband and I share the chance to pat Grace's back and inhale the milky scent of new baby. Emily's brothers hear the baby whimper and sit with Emily as she feeds and changes and bathes her little girl. Even though it brings such an ache to our hearts to know it is only for a little while, we each love her as much as we possibly can.

Emily swaddles Grace in blankets of blue and pink. She sleeps with Grace in her arms. This birthmother makes the very best of their limited time together. Emily rocks her baby, rubs her baby, loves her baby fully. She is the very best mother she can be for that short time.

In their last moment together, when Emily cradles Grace in her arms and then slowly passes her baby over to her new mother, she does so with a smile. We all, Emily, Jeannie, that new mother and I, stand together and cherish the shared love of this baby, our miracle.

After the baby leaves, we will each become separate stones in our grief. Emily most of all. But for now she smiles as she says her parenting is done. Now it is this new mother's turn. Emily doesn't want to hurt Grace with tears. She doesn't want to make this new mother sad for her. We each stand stoically, witness to this couple's joy, our daughter's loss.

Emily's tears are shed only after Grace's new mother and father have gone. I stand in the hallway, feeling the weight of empty arms. I can hear the muffled

59

sounds of crying behind closed doors from every corner of our home. And there is nothing I can do to offer comfort. Not now. We are each too raw with our grief.

The days following Grace's leaving are quiet and sad. But slowly, just as we gathered to share in this baby's love, we now reach out and gather together to offer Emily comfort.

It takes time. One of the hardest things we can teach our children is how to live despite grief. But, as a family, we do. Slowly, our sadness and Emily's sorrow are diminished, replaced with love from the distance of this adoption.

This is the story of a birthmother who placed her baby for adoption because she is too young. It is the story of shared kinship, that we've learned doesn't really end through adoption. Like the surface of water broken by a stone, it ripples out into the world to touch mothers and daughters, fathers, brothers, and sisters. This is the story of a unique kinship that forms a family.

It is the story of a baby who was loved and is loved. She brings joy each day to the family who raises her. She brings joy to her family of origin. We know she is happy. We know she is safe. She is loved.

This is also the story of a girl-woman who gave birth and knows sorrow. She will grow up and love again. These days she has dreams. She makes plans for the day when she is ready to have a family of her own.

This is a short story about a baby's birth, but sad as it may seem, it doesn't really end that way. It doesn't really end at all.

Emily's is a story that began with love; it is about waiting for a birth. It is laden with broken hearts and sad moments. But it is also a story that continues to form joy out of love. Imagine Grace turning into a little girl who knows she was cherished from the first. Imagine my own daughter smiling, knowing she made the right choice, when she receives annual pictures of Grace with her parents, playing, living, loving. Imagine Emily's tranquility as she places those photos onto the creamy pages of photo albums, her voice a melody of lullabies.

This is the story of an end. But it is also a story of beginning again.

8

Out of the Woods

Pierre Laroche

The first call is a dance. I already know, but that is little comfort in this awkward business of announcing death; the message resists slipping from our throats. It is as if death itself demands our attention, shaking us anew with each mention. He wonders how much more he has to say. I know, I feel what he wonders…

"Your receptionist called the office…I'm so sorry; how is your wife?"

"Fine. Yeah. Thanks?" he utters, preoccupied but relieved at not having to continue.

"Is there anything we can do?" And the dance continues, difficult and predetermined. The truth is, I am relieved not to have to hear him struggle through the chronology. I am relieved not to have to hear him pull off being the strong one. My wife and other women in the office will ask me for details and will shake their heads in amazement that I don't have them. They will wonder aloud what men talk about. I cringe at the thought that this will become another of the gender litanies that are trotted out at parties: Men are from Mars blah blah blah.

The truth is, I am relieved because I understand all I need to understand when I hear the slow and deliberate pace of his voice. I know all I need to know as confused needs flow like unintoned questions from his lips. He is alone and needs my help for something, logistical problems; he knows he will get the help, but for the rest he will be alone. He would prefer to be with his wife struggling through this death of their child, through this reality, rather than the news of it.

It is enough that I hear the alienation, the deep waters of comfortless remembrance seeping to the surface. For moments at a time, you can lose yourself in the world's patterns, but sooner or later you are alone with all of it.

I know what it is like to be alone with your lover, reminded again and again of the tenuous thread that binds us to this world and to each other.

So, I don't ask.

Another friend of mine writes courageously about his wife's miscarriage. I am swept away by the moment the tiny, still body rests lovingly on the belly of its mother. The idea of pregnancy ending with death, of the womb as tomb, of the two of them huddled in love and misery around the body of a child that will never grow with them. What happened to them happens to many, as he writes eloquently, but the moment is so intense with fear and pain that we wince and want to ignore it. And so as a society we deny the scar that makes us shudder, and make freakish the need to do anything but forget the child that never was.

I have been to her grave with him several times. It seems that the hospital normally disposes of the tissue, but he and his wife insisted on burying her on their land in the mountains. Even now, years after, I see him pause near her grave; she is with him now as she was on that autumn day when he precisely carved the earth for her. She is with his wife now as she was when she sewed the funerary dress of doll proportions. And while it seems exaggerated, in a very real way she is with all of us: all of us who have visited and had his oldest take us to the grave to introduce us to his sister; all of us who have heard his wife tell the story of her still birth as she does about the three live births; all of us who have noticed the swing set placed not far away or that his parents keep flowers on the grave.

Regardless of who she might have been, through this family I see how life and death work together, how grace comes from struggling into pain. It is a fire-forged truth, fashioned out of desperate need and hope: our life is nothing more than what happens to us and those we love.

Out of the Woods

I hear on National Public Radio some men complaining about how they are expected to coach their wives through birth. They discuss the undue stress that has been put on them, the fainting at the sign of blood, the general discomfort they must endure for reasons of mere political correctness in the 90s, the general nastiness of their wives during labor. It is amusing to hear these guys imply that this moment revolves chiefly around their own efforts. They sound so afraid that something might go wrong, or worse, that something might reflect badly on them. I feel sorry for them and all they willingly lose as they forsake the opportunity of a new beginning for a vinyl seat in someone else's hospital.

My first child was like a journey through the desert. We read the books, kept the log, listened to heartbeats that quickly connected us to him. But nothing prepares a person for the abrahamian task of moving your family from the two of you, to us three. It is a flustering and humble tumble into biology, management and spirituality.

From the first contraction to the birth 36 hours later, we are in the weather. At first it is the unsettling pain, the stretching and thunderous clouds at the horizon. By evening the storm is on the edge of town, the sky darkens and the wind blows the yard a mess. In the early morning, the rain and storm are upon us, dashing us this way and that. My wife has visions, talks to the long dead, sits in our shower stall barely big enough for someone who isn't pregnant. As the lightning strikes and thunderclaps bear down on us, the hour approaches. The fatigue and restless waiting are over: in one moment, I am holding her as she pushes; in the next, we cradle his glistening body to us, selfish in the glow.

"Breathe," I command the child, tenderly rubbing his ruddy torso with my hand. "Breathe, baby, breathe." Even now, the hope, the desire, the vulnerability of those words rings within me. Tears still come to our eyes as we remember how he chirped auspiciously and nuzzled into her breast.

What remains is the power of it all. The shaky realization that there is no controlling much of it, you are at its mercy. Often birth is romanticized, but the glaring wonder for me is not the gauzy, almost erotic, images of a Madonna and child. I am drawn to the unpredictability of a moment that predictably delivers sweat and blood. It is at once traumatic and awe-inspiring, an event that feels so essential to my understanding of my wife and myself that I hardly remember how I saw things before her labor.

I remember in the long hours of early morning, when the night was especially dark and the hopes of a quick labor had long since passed, a frightening reality emerged. As her contractions rippled involuntarily across her belly and her pain was both undeniable and unstoppable, I was alone with her, completely alone. There was nothing to do but wait and watch…wait and hold her hand as a vague comfort against the biological winds that will always be greater than any one of us. I am not practiced at this and it is disappointing that there isn't more for me to do but sit and witness. Sometime later, after the birth, I articulate this frustration, and she says it is all she wanted.

And maybe for the first time we were really married, really together in something. And while there is this unfathomable joy in receiving the new babe in its first minutes of extra-utero existence, there is also an amazing sorrow in recognizing that there is nothing much you can do for your wife or child. The world, in all its splendor and crystalline precision, will have its way with your children, your parents, your lover, and there is nothing much you can do…but hold her hand.

I looked forward to the arid march of my second son's gestation. We braced ourselves for a drawn out labor and all of the attending emotions of frustration and impatience. While her labor built all night, we watched a movie, slept relatively well, and settled in to witness the drama unfold.

On Thanksgiving Day, only five hours after I awoke, he emerged, his cord firmly wrapped around his neck, purple, without pulse or breath.

"Breathe," I beg as we try to rub mucous out of and air into his lungs. He looks dead, or soon dead. And all the discussions we have had about the safety of home birth and the fear of mishap ring loud in my ears.

"He's OK," I lie and she looks more worried than I have ever seen.

"Is it a boy or a girl?" she asks.

"Don't worry about that now," orders the mid-wife, "we're just trying to get it breathing."

Out of the Woods

We have rationalized that babies die, that part of the bargain in being active in our children's birth is the possibility that things might go awry, that life and death are separated by a fragile thread. We wanted to witness that thread, so that life might seem more special, more a part of us, more alive. With friends who have felt that thread snap, we were aware that death exists just beyond the periphery. We understood, if only intellectually, that death is never so far off from the overpowering exhilaration of life.

But now, as my son seems to be dying in my hands, I know and fear we are approaching that obvious intersection. Now, there is nothing theoretical about it.

"OK, we've got to get this baby breathing. People, talk to your baby... Mama, talk to your baby!" orders the mid-wife again.

"Breathe," I utter flatly, impatiently.

"But is it a boy or a girl?" she pleads this time.

"OK, Mama, it's a boy."

I raise him, purplish and prone, to his mother.

Empathetic, she looks at his limp body; and with what must have been his final ounce of energy, he stares back at the sound of her voice.

"Breathe, Dante, breathe," she coaxes.

Maybe for more seconds than he has been alive, he stares at his mother. And slowly, as he witnesses his mother for the first time, his heart and lungs begin their rhythmic pumping. She says often that it was in those moments, as the thread stretched to breaking, that Dante decided to stay with us, to give our family a whirl.

And more than ever, my elation and sorrow are premised on the same, simple realization: these beautiful people, all these beautiful people pass through my life, capture my heart, look to me for strength, and all I can offer them is the knowledge that I have no answers, no real power, no influence in the universe. I will stand with them but all I can really offer is my hand.

And with all of this, with the pain and the hope and the mystery of all of this...we sit down grateful with our hours old infant, the midwives, and a neighbor, to eat the day's meal.

A colleague of mine spent a decade trying to be a mother. It was difficult to watch her not able to share in such an obvious and predictable way. Eventually, after years of fertility treatments, she was pregnant. She and her husband were overjoyed; this was the moment they had dreamed of, the opportunity to set right what they felt was missing. My wife was pregnant at exactly the same moment, and I remember that joy. I remember feeling my wife's belly for signs of my child, for signs of me, in the alchemy of gestation. I remember the goofy conversations with the fetus that, according to the books, didn't yet have ears to hear me. "Come out," I would invite. "Come out and play."

And so it was crushing when my colleague lost her baby in the first trimester. Death is always hard, especially the death of children. And this was hard because it seemed so unfair. She told me once that she found it difficult to face the fertile teenagers in our classes, because it seemed wasted on them. She was describing more than disappointment; it was a crisis of faith. Beyond the selfish desire to shape the world according to a plan, the problem with death is that it feels so personal. The pains of loss and the weight of feeling that the universe is predisposed against us overwhelm. It's difficult not to get angry when bad things seem to happen to good people, especially when we are the good, the abandoned, the righteous. She and her husband lost parents in the same year as they lost parenthood. And I could see that despite the brave face, it was an enormous effort for her to do anything but retreat into her home and marriage, and escape the reminders of all that was lost.

Perhaps a year later, as I was feeling the first stages of fatherhood, I spoke explicitly with her about it. "I don't mean to pry," I said awkwardly, "but you seem so positive these past few months. Are you feeling better?"

"Not really," she replied. "It's still hard to understand all of it, but I guess its not so consuming anymore."

What I saw was a confidence, a directness that she had seemed to lack before. Where before she would opt for silence, now she spoke up, voiced her concerns, participated in the fray. It felt as if she had turned a corner.

"I guess my problem was that I saw all that was happening to me as a tragedy. It's hard to live in a tragedy. One day I realized that while it was awful, it wasn't tragic, it was just life. I think it helps me to recognize that I have had a lot of life happening recently."

And that feels like a key, recognizing what's happening is special; it's life. Tragedy is a kind of self-indulgent fantasy that presumes that the universe has it out for us; it is a terrible burden to shoulder. Pain in life is what it is, part of an adventure, maybe not wonderful, but part of it nonetheless. It is no small task to embrace the life we have, rather than wish for one we don't. It is the essence of grace.

At the foot of his hospital bed, even before he dies, the pain of my father-in-law's death is everywhere around me, my wife's tired and red eyes, the quiet slump of his girlfriend's posture. He draws in air through a gaping mouth that makes him look like a fish out of water; he flops on the sand or the dock or the sidewalk, a stylized cartoon of some other species' suffering. Despite his 66 years, he has become the sound of his lips: pah…pah…pah. In the abstract, the popping comforts, like the ticking of a clock or the crackle of a radio. But as distant and beautiful as it sometimes sounds, I know that this rhythm punctuates the pregnant grief in the room. And so this is how it goes for the next few hours, this oscillation between the moments of his dying—amazing and brilliant unto themselves—and the routine remembering that I am part of a family who will lose someone today.

His breathing is rhythmic and slowing. I sit quietly, trying to focus on nothing, failing, and feeling my own breath. Mine is not his rhythm. He seems in sync with the flashing light of his IV monitor; but no, he is slowing. His labored gape drifts from the light to the time between the flashes and back again. Occasionally, his breath pauses entirely; his girlfriend stops her crossword and I my writing. Just as mysteriously, the breath returns; his breathing is an overloaded gear making its labored and final revolutions. What he knows, I do not know; the experts claim that the renal and liver failure has caused toxins to leak into his blood and that what we refer to as mind has been dead for hours. The breathing and sighing now is just a reflex, the final struggle heaped on top of weeks of pain. What he feels, or sees, or wants, I do not know. I am comforted by the thought that he is past that now, past the painful details and the worry and the second-guessing. He is becoming his gears.

Of course, he is not becoming his gears, he has always been his gears; it's just that now, there is no energy for anything else. Like barred teeth or a bloody wound, the only thing new is my seeing it; the teeth and muscle and bone have always been there. But somehow, because it is her father, or because I've never really seen him before, all of this is fresh and raw. It is shocking how much of a struggle dying really is, how difficult it is even for the gears to let go, and it is hard to watch. I remember my wife laboring through childbirth and feeling that I was witnessing not who she was, but rather what she is. Up until that point, I found it difficult to reconcile the objective and subjective feelings I had for her, somehow imagining that the objective was dehumanizing. Then somewhere in the fatigue and collapse after the birth, I remember understanding that she is both, or rather that she is my understanding of her gears as well as my understanding of her story. What a relief, as if I was seeing her for the first time, fresh, without a censor, without blame and worry, nestling our son.

So as tempted as I am to deny the waxy translucence of his skin now—implying yet again his impending disappearance—I can't deny or regret his gears. His story may slip first, leaving him naked, yellowed and ashen and stiff and smelly and heaving for air, but he is all of it. And so am I, all of it. I watch the rhythm halt, and I mutter, "Good work," and everyone knows. I take a deep, deliberate breath, move to hug her, fresh, without worry, as if it was the very first time.

Some weekends ago, a family not so distant from mine lost a son. Struck by a train going 40 miles an hour, two very loveable teenage brothers find themselves on the spur of fate. One, the driver, walks away with minor injuries and the scar of a lifetime. The other dies instantly. It is not unlike my parents' nightmares that I so easily dismissed, and that I now find haunting the shadows of my imagination. Once I was drawn to the messiness of this border between life and death so I could feel more alive; now I know that when I don't see it, I'm just fooling myself.

At the table some days later, after hearing a revision of this essay, my wife confesses, "I never told you this before, but I knew something was wrong with

Dante, and I prayed every day that he would be born alive." She breathes heavy, as I do now in the rawness of it. "While I worried about him dying in birth, now I realize that his life can end at any moment, that birth was the least of his worries." Another pause.

"We are not out of the woods yet," she finishes. Of course, she's being kind. She knows that I want there to be woods that we can safely get beyond. The truth is, there are no woods and we'll never be out of them. Quieted by fortune and loss, we sit in our kitchen trying as best we can to face this familiar uncertainty.

9

The Mantra of Acceptance

Anne Winterich

I have been on bed rest for six weeks and in the hospital for the last eight days and when I will be able to leave is anybody's guess. Had I known eight weeks ago that a trip for Christmas to see my parents would extend into a two-month stay fraught with constant dread and pain, I would have stayed home. But fly across the country we did—my husband, my five-year-old daughter, and my 27 weeks pregnant self—California to Georgia, a five day trip that turned horrifying the night before we were due to fly home when a routine two a.m. bathroom call suddenly turned into hemorrhaging. I was rushed to the emergency room to discover that the partial placenta previa, a condition in which the placenta covers the cervical os, that had shown up on my 18 week sonogram was, in fact, still present. My doctor had assured me chances of this were so remote that he had put me on no restrictions. I exercised. I had intercourse. I flew across the country, completely oblivious that the placenta previa was still a part of my pregnancy.

Hindsight is 20/20. A quick sonogram before flying would have alleviated two months of hell. That my vision is perfect only in looking back infuriates me. These days with the future so fuzzy, I can only focus on what has passed. It hurts too much to squint into my blurry days to come—days filled with endless hours stuck in a hospital bed, the view from my window a first story flat roof courtyard interspersed with pipes and ducts and filters, a fast food drink cup and straw, a broken corner of Styrofoam insulation, a plastic bag. Endless hours broken only by a steady rotation of doctors and nurses and technicians who poke and prod and push and peer. Any bleeding? Spotting? Contractions? Feveracheschills? Swelling? Baby moving okay?

A quiet routine consists of a 7 a.m. breakfast. Between 8 and 9 a.m., my doctors visit (see questions above), shift changes, new nurse comes in and repeats every action and question of doctors who just left room but has the added task of giving me my Colace pill (to help bowel movements along), which I politely refuse.

An hour or two later, the tech comes in to take my vitals and also checks my blood sugar level because, along with everything else, I've developed gestational diabetes and must get two insulin shots a day. Next, she helps me into a wheelchair to take me for my daily Non-Stress Test, at which I am hooked up to a fetal monitor that measures baby's heartbeat and my contractions (or lack of, hopefully) for 30 minutes

Just before lunch, my nurse delivers another pill I mustn't refuse. This one is to keep contractions at bay. Sometimes she remembers to bring my a.m. snack —a pint of skim milk and half a mystery meat sandwich on white bread with a tiny packet of mustard and no knife to spread it. Because I am shaky with hunger, I eat it.

11:30 brings lunch. I have the privilege of choosing my meals (from a set diabetic menu of course). Entrees are decorated with a sprig of parsley and a cherry tomato and consist of meat or cottage cheese and fruit. Starches include grits, a choice with every meal, mashed potatoes, white rice, white dinner roll, or corn bread. (I'm amazed I don't need the Colace.) Dessert choices are depressing: Jell-o, canned fruit, vanilla wafers, ginger snaps. Every day, I circle the least of these evils, gingersnaps. With each request, I get back a polite note at the top of my meal ticket which reads: "Some of the items you selected have been changed to comply with your diet orders." Hence the jello. I consider writing back and asking why gingersnaps are a choice in the first place if they don't meet my "diet orders" but decide to be nice. Free Foods is actually a heading, as if it will make me feel better about all the lousy options above it, and consists of salt, pepper, sugar substitute, iced tea, coffee, creamer, and Crystal lite lemonade. I circle all of these one day to get back at the kitchen for the gingersnap thing.

Meanwhile, my husband Dan and my daughter Madeleine have arrived and we talk and color or watch *Dragon Tales.* I'm not much fun these days, but one morning in a burst of creativity we haven't felt in weeks, Madeleine ties string up around the room and I cut out little clothes from paper towels and we hang them on the lines like laundry blowing in a fresh breeze.

When they leave I nap if possible, but more checking of vitals and swelling and baby's heartbeat and IV flushes inevitably keep that from happening. I just want to sleep continuously, worry and guilt free, until baby can be born without risk.

Dinner heralds a small blip in the monotony of the day when, in addition to the tech taking my vitals and blood sugar, she measures my pee, which I have reluctantly "collected" in a bowl that fits over the toilet seat. I refused to do this for several days and got away with it, but then the doctor granted my request to drop my fluid drip so I feel obligated to pee in a bowl for her. Kitchen staff, the only staff that consistently knocks and waits for an answer, comes to clear my tray. It's the saddest part of the day; too early to go to sleep, nothing interesting on TV, Dan and Madeleine long gone. I'm emotionally spent from worrying baby is not going to make it, feeling guilty that I wasn't more proactive about my prenatal care, and wishing I was home.

Every two hours from now until morning, the tech wakes me up to take my vitals. When breakfast is finally delivered, I offer up a silent prayer of thanks that I am one day closer to the end of this nightmare I wish I'd seen coming and been able to avoid.

Hindsight allows me to see myself refusing to buy into Dr. R.'s cavalier attitude about my placenta previa, me taking the precautions he should have advised: pelvic rest, bed rest, and most certainly, no flights 3,000 freakin' miles across the country 27 weeks pregnant. I see now I should have insisted on a sonogram before flying to see if my previa had corrected itself, should have asked "what if?" questions before traveling, such as: What if, out of nowhere, in the middle of the night before we're set to fly home, I wake up to find blood covering the sheets of my bed and I have to be rushed to the emergency room?

Hindsight allows me to see the consuming worries about the baby, Madeleine, Dan, our home, our business, Madeleine's schooling, money, and the logistics of suddenly being stranded 3,000 miles from home in an unfamiliar city, life as we have known it completely on hold until baby is born and we can all fly back to California. Best case scenario is home by end of February. Very wishful thinking. Worst case, home at the end of March after having been gone for three months. My 20/20 hindsight flashes constantly a beacon of warning: Err on the side of caution! Stay close to home during a pregnancy!

I can rage with clear hindsight all I want, but it doesn't change one thing. The only certainty of this situation is that I am not in control. My body acts of its own accord, the doctors react in response to that, and baby will come when she comes. I can hope for things, but hoping these last seven weeks has been a constant exercise in futility. And yet, I continue to hope. It is all I can do.

I hope baby will be okay. I hope the bleeding will stop, that I can fly home, that time will pass quickly. Hope Madeleine won't be traumatized by all of this. Hope I just start bleeding profusely and have to have an emergency c-section to stop this endless wait on tenterhooks. Hope amniocentesis shows baby's developed lungs. Hope I can deliver early. Hope baby is healthy. Hope baby and I are strong enough to fly home immediately. Hope. Hope. Hope.

But the only responses to my hoping so far are several "episodes," as the doctors refer to them. Like they're made for daytime TV drama. Anytime, anywhere, no pattern or prediction, I start to bleed, each episode more intense than the last. If "home" (i.e. house we're renting indefinitely, located across the street from my parents and 30 minutes from hospital), we drop everything and drive fast in car to hospital. We do this three times before doctors decide I am too far away from the hospital to remain at home. I'm admitted for the duration of my pregnancy and, once there, an "episode" means buzz nurse, drop everything, drive fast in my bed down hallway to labor and delivery. Feel sick to my stomach due to panic. Call Dan who drops everything and drives fast to hospital. Pray very hard.

Nurses check vitals, strap me into fetal monitor, insert two IV's, one for fluids and meds, the other for possible blood transfusion, draw blood from arm. Doctor arrives and does a pelvic exam, always comments on the number and size of clots passing. Like I want to know. Listen for baby's heartbeat: hear it, feel relief. Cross fingers and toes for contractions to stop. Starving but go without food in case an emergency c-section is necessary. Must pee in a bedpan and lie on labor bed until a) I stabilize and can be moved back to my room (this takes hours) or b) I get rushed to the operating room.

The benefits of a) are baby gets more time to develop in my womb, thereby decreasing risks and complications at birth and I get to return to a comfortable bed, unhook monitor, and pee in a toilet.

The benefits of b) are double-edged. Baby is born, thereby ending this particular wild ride. No more bleeding, IV's, monitors, bedpans, needles, bad food, or hospital gowns. But she's premature and likely to have complications. With scenario b), I trade one set of worries for another.

Never in my wildest imaginings did I envision any part of these last seven weeks. I am supposed to be home right now ordering new carpet for the girls' room, buying a dresser with a changing table top, assembling the cradle and sewing a bumper pad for it, pulling down bins of baby clothes I've saved. Making stacks of tiny onesies. I am supposed to be home cherishing these last months alone with Madeleine, gently preparing her for the many ways her life will change with a baby in the house, babying her just a little bit longer before she must give up center stage.

I can't help feeling I'm being tested by some greater force, God, whatever, but I haven't studied for the exam. I don't know the material or the rules. Do other people in similar situations? Is it okay to feel angry with a doctor who's human and capable of mistakes? How do I rectify feeling that this situation sucks beyond belief and the fact that it could be far worse? How do I forgive myself for worrying about me too?

I hear through my nurse that another woman from California has been admitted for pregnancy complications and, like me, will be here, probably for weeks, until her baby is born and healthy enough to fly home. The nurse says she's a "real hoot." How does she do that, hoot her way through worries and anger and guilt?

Someone please teach me the Mantra of Acceptance so that I can just *be* these coming weeks. I don't think I can get there on my own and yet I don't want anyone telling me what to feel thankful for or that this will all be over soon, that the baby will be okay. I find it impossible to believe these truths. E-mails that advise lots of journal writing and sipping of tea and relishing complete inactivity makes me want to throw the computer across the room. There are days when I am so consumed by anxiety and anger that I hear these statements only as platitudes rather than the messages of support and encouragement and love intended.

Perhaps I should go back to hoping. Hope my 20/20 hindsight fades, forcing me to focus on the future. What's required to accept it, I just don't know. Does anyone out there? Throw me a line.

Postscript...

My baby girl was born by emergency c-section on February 14th, five weeks early, a real fighter who, despite days of breathing troubles and severe jaundice in intensive care, was able to check out of the hospital and fly home to California a week after her birth. Her name is Thea Colette. Of Greek origins, Thea means a gift of God. Colette (French) means victorious in battle. She is currently a happy and healthy one-year-old handful.

Thea's birth, which, according to my doctors, took all of 20 minutes, was, in many ways, the least significant event of this whole experience. I woke the morning of the 14th hemorrhaging badly. The c-section stopped the bleeding, ended the placenta previa as well as the gestational diabetes, and safely brought my girl into the world. Despite being an emergency, it was fairly routine. I even got a bikini incision. I was knocked out cold for it. When I woke 45 minutes later, I had a baby girl and Dan was there holding my hand, smiling. What did it matter that I needed two blood transfusions the next day due to the amount of blood I'd lost or that I couldn't hold Thea for the first day because she was hooked up to so many tubes and wires and needles? She was going to be fine and so was I and suddenly the future looked brilliantly clear.

10

La Promesa de Esperanza

Noemi Martinez

I was four months pregnant, laying on the bed with my fist against my belly, hoping that I would feel some movement inside.

I drank caffeine, ate spicy food, sipped ice water. For days, I waited for a flutter, those butterfly-rumbling sensations that signal a presence.

I had been choked and beaten a few days earlier in my mom's backyard, by someone I had once loved, the father of the baby I was carrying. I remember being on the floor and my older brother and younger brother, along with my mother, were immobilized behind us, watching the scene unfold. Surely, their arms and legs were cemented down, their vocal cords severed—because they didn't protect me or shield me as strong hands worked their way around my neck. Days later, I thought maybe these cells and tiny heart were no longer beating, and I was alone again. Finally, I went to the doctor and was reassured when I heard the *thump thump thump* on the baby monitor.

I knew I was pregnant at two weeks. But I was barely living. I was caring for my three-year-old son River, recently separated from his father, and trying to make ends meet. For a long time, I didn't feel pregnant: my belly never grew; there were no congratulatory hugs.

My own deeply religious father was outraged that I was separated from my husband and pregnant with another man's baby. Marriage was sacred and I had committed sin upon sin. Getting pregnant with another man's baby, living with someone that wasn't my husband. What had happened to my religious upbringing and the years of Bible classes? he wondered. I told him that my new boyfriend, let's call him "Joe," was hitting me when he'd get angry. He responded that it was God's will and I should pray about it. When Joe broke up with me and left me when I was three months pregnant, it was punishment for not walking the straight path. Dad stopped speaking to me eventually, and I guess God has long been silent.

I moved into my mom's house because I couldn't afford the rent by myself and the living room became our bedroom. One day after I came back from the park with River, Joe was there. He had been my brother's best friend and they treated him like one of the family. Mom asked me to leave so I wouldn't cause a scene. Betrayal doesn't cover the way I felt. He was like a son to her, she said. Even though he didn't want to be in the baby's life and had broken up with me when I was three months pregnant, she would stand next to him.

For those nine months, it seemed time stopped and I couldn't breathe. This was surely the result of me being a bad daughter, a bad person, a bad mother, not praying enough—always too emotional, always asking too many questions, never settling.

I went to the monthly appointments alone and once, when they drew blood, I fainted. Waited for it to pass as I lay on an examination table; waited for it to pass because there was no one to call. I stopped eating and lost weight. In Spanish, we call it *ánimo*, meaning spirit or enthusiasm, and I was certainly lacking *ánimo*.

It never failed—Joe would show up at my mom's house. I couldn't tell him to leave, and he never asked about the baby. I went to my mom's bedroom when he came over to hang out with my brother and sister. Sometimes the story unfolded again, me on the floor of the living room, being kicked, with my sister in the kitchen. Once when I was six months pregnant, after a call from my sister, I was removed in handcuffs by the police because I was causing a disturbance. The police did not ask about the domestic abuse.

Joe and my family would watch movies or play games. I would go driving with River or lay on my mom's bed, singing to the little bright light growing inside of me, waiting for him to leave.

No one was happy. No one acknowledged me. I remember feeling like the pregnant teenager everyone blamed. A zine I put out while I was pregnant read, "There is no comfort in my suffering and I have no one and no where to go, no one to turn to. I have become nothing and no one to everybody. I have become no one to them, I was in pieces, and they turned me away. Live with it. Live with it. Live with it."

It seems like for the nine months I was carrying Esperanza, the labor and the delivery, I was mentally preparing myself for being the single parent I was going to be. I sought strength and solace while I was pregnant, often going to sleep looking at the trees swaying, silently, rhythmically. Fighting the depression that was sinking me. I would look at the trees and wonder how they endured all weather, standing tall. Others were damaged and might be bent or have branches no longer growing, but they still stood firm, their roots firmly planted.

Still at my mom's house, I slept on my mom's futon-turned-bed with River sleeping by my side. He would often sing and talk to my growing stomach. There was a box fan on the windowsill that blew hot air in and rearranged the dust. I scoured garage sales, thrift stores and *segundas* for baby clothes. I asked my cousins and aunts for their used walkers and swings. I pawned just about everything I had leftover from the separation for a new stroller and baby carrier. We were set.

But there were mice in the refrigerator. The little house mom was renting was literally falling apart, leaving big gaping holes in the walls. We figured this is how they sneaked in. We started putting our food in plastic containers. The walls were caving in and the heat unbearable. In the laundry room, we saw the sunlight streaming in. The toilet was sinking. I tried not to cry in front of River. I even prayed.

Little Esperanza was two weeks behind schedule, but I didn't want to rush her arrival and told the doctor as long as everything was okay, I didn't want to be induced. I talked and sang to her, letting her know she would be loved. I wrote her letters, saying my heart was big enough to love both her and her brother River. It was the end of June when the contractions started, 101 degrees in hot sunny South Texas—we were in the *canicula*, the hottest part of the summer. With sweat beading on my forehead and trickling down my legs, I didn't realize I started to bleed. With no pain, my water broke. It was happening; the climax had started.

I was alone in my thoughts and in myself for most of the labor. My memory gets hazy at this point. I was impressed with the room with its rocking chair and two nightstands, and I compared it to the place this baby would make her home. My mom drove me and we put River in his car seat, next to the bag I'd packed for the baby and me. River was there with me for a while before it got intense, and then he went home with my mom. I asked if he was excited that his sister was coming. He looked towards my belly and said to Esperanza, "Don't stay in there, come out already!"

When they wheeled me in for an emergency c-section after 14 hours, the attendants, nurses, and doctors talked to each other as if I wasn't there. I'd wanted a natural birth, but River had been born with complications and a collapsed lung, spending weeks in the neonatal intensive care, so I was ready to relinquish responsibility to someone else—if only for a few hours. The doctors and nurses asked each other who was with me. "Is someone going to be here with her? Should we wait?" Finally, I told them not to wait. There was no one.

I said nothing when they pulled Esperanza out. In the shiny reflection on the overhead medical lamp, her long and lanky body slithered. I watched as they separated my insides. Did they know I could see everything? She cried the sweet song I had waited for. Unlike River, who couldn't breathe when he was born, her lungs were clean and forceful. As they wheeled me out, the doctor said she was concerned about me. I had not said anything when I held Esperanza. "I'm all right," I reassured her, "just tired."

Over the next few years, I worked more than I slept. I was continuously sick. Night shifts. I left my mom's and started living on my own. There were countless court dates. Eventually, my family came to see negative space as what it really was—a black hole—and Joe was no longer welcomed in their home.

Esperanza became the renewal process. What happens after a storm. She is the embodiment of dancing light. Along with my son River, we have formed this tight balance of part comedy act, part creative family, part super heroes.

Labor Pains and Birth Stories

This birth of myself
into who I am now
was a process
of layers being built and torn down,
 reconstructed.
Pieced together now,
I'm a collage.
Spackled together with heavy resin.
Parts mismatched with faded paper of facts, data,
            dates, and numbers.
Glued with bone and blood and tough tissue.
What once was broken, made whole.
Ready now—not perfect, but together.
There are holes, scratches,
dots that can't be connected.
There are gaps
and questions to come
I don't know how to answer yet.

11

Had Baby. Bring Coffee

Ariel Gore

Paternity meant nothing to the ancients. They attributed conception to inadvertently swallowing insects, to eating beans, or to the wind.

We've opted for a friend's donor sperm, inseminated with an oral medicine syringe.

Eight months later, the contractions start. Every 20 minutes, then every 15 minutes, every ten minutes, then every 20 again. Most nights I can't sleep. August days pass slow like whispered dreams. The heat. Sunlight stretching into the night. The contractions don't hurt, exactly, but they distract me from sleep and work. I'm glad it wasn't like this with my first baby. If I'd never been in labor before, I'd be fooled.

My first baby. Maia. 17 1/2 years ago. I was homeless for the first half of the pregnancy, only gained ten or 15 pounds. I'd forgotten so much about those sweet traveling months of my late adolescence, but now this second pregnancy reminds me.

"I keep thinking about Italy," I tell Fabulosa.

"Maybe you're going to have the baby tonight?" she whispers.

"Maybe," I say, but the contractions aren't that intense.

As Maia packs up to head south for college, my uterus tightens and relaxes, tightens and relaxes. I hope the baby will come early to meet his sister before she has to go. 38 weeks. 39 weeks. Strangers heckle me on the street: "When are you going to have that baby?"

The car is full of Maia's shoes, but I'm still pregnant.

I clean the blinds. Fabulosa paints the bathroom. We are both nesting.

I listen to Giuditta Tornetta's *Joyful Birth* CD, try to learn self-hypnosis for a "natural and painless childbirth." At first it seems almost too cheesy, but I listen every day, fall asleep as I listen, and I start to feel the fear and old trauma peel away. It's been a long time since I had Maia. And it wasn't all joyful or painless. I felt scared. My boyfriend was drunk. I couldn't understand the doctors. They tied me down to a metal table with leather straps, cut an episiotomy the young midwives stare at now. "Where did you get that?" they want to know. They squint.

"They were still cutting episiotomies like that 17 years ago in Europe," the older midwife assures.

My body is a museum, an ancient map.

At the "resource center" where I got my free pregnancy test, the counselor asked if I was married. No, I told her. She gave me a pamphlet that kindly informed me: *The Only Safe Sex is No Sex Until Faithful Married Sex.* If she only knew. My immaculate lesbian conception.

The average pregnancy lasts 41 weeks, but I'm getting nervous now.

Maia was born the day she was due. It was wintertime.

"Boys are always late," a grocery checker tells me. I linger in the air-conditioned store.

I'm three and a half centimeters dilated, but the contractions refuse to intensify. I've tried everything—walking and drinking oil, Flamenco dancing and visualization, a self-imposed zine deadline and spicy spinach curry. Fabulosa places acupuncture needles in my ankles, encourages our son along.

Uncle Donor sends daily text messages. *Any news?*

Walter at the post office shakes his head when he sees me. "When are you going to have that baby?"

The midwives talk about induction. After Labor Day, we'll consider it. But I want to wait.

Two days before the lunar eclipse I go to the co-op, intent on finding an elixir. I decide on a big bottle of organic pineapple juice and a bright red herbal tea infusion.

Had Baby. Bring Coffee

The day before Maia was born, a shopkeeper in the tiny Tuscan village where I lived invited me into the back of her shop and gave me two silver and coral charms. "One for you, one for the baby," she told me. "To keep you from the evil eye."

The writing teacher Tom Spanbauer tells his students to slow down the narrative when an object changes hands in a story, to linger in the moment of exchange, because right here and now in the story, energy is changing hands.

Fabulosa hands me a jar of pomegranate juice. "To keep you hydrated," she says.

In old iconographic paintings, the Virgin Mary sometimes holds Persephone's pomegranate—to symbolize her authority over birth and death.

Now Fabulosa and I drive out to the edge of town for a student's book signing and reception. She's sick from cancer and bone thin from chemo, but my student beams. A book! She has written and published this real book. We eat cream puffs and all the other guests marvel at my size. I've gained 50 pounds this time.

Maia calls from Los Angeles. She is settling into her apartment. Classes start on Tuesday. "And the baby? When will he come?"

When I was in labor with her, a giant clock hung on the wall over my bed. The hands on that thing didn't move, the face of the clock just got bigger and bigger until all the numbers were blurred and unreadable. I was underwater, breathing somehow through the blue, far away from my drunken boyfriend, far from those nurses who just wanted to yell at me.

On our way back from the book signing now, Fabulosa spots a bright, round UFO in the darkening summer sky. We follow it for a while, watching. It's not a plane, not the moon, not a searchlight. It moves closer to the earth, looks so solid. And then—*blink*—it's gone. Nina Hagen saw a UFO before her daughter, Cosma Shiva, was born. There was a little recording studio on board.

Back home now and into the night, the same old regular/irregular contractions, but I have a weird sense of dejavu: I've dreamed this night before. *No matter—to sleep.* At 1:30 I get up to pee, gush a good leak of amniotic fluid. I figure this is it—has to be—but it's happened before. *Either this is it or it isn't.*

"Poor little Gypsy baby," the nurses said when Maia was born.

They didn't know about the charms I had in my back pack, didn't know how far we'd traveled, didn't know how far we'd go.

In that song, *On & On*, Eryka Badu says she was born with three dollars and six dimes. What she means is this: She was born whole, she was not broke.

I putter around the house for an hour, snap a picture of myself looking crazy, finally wake Fabulosa. "I don't know if I'm in labor or not," I tell her. "How about let's go to the store and get some fizzy water?"

I pace the aisles in the fluorescent glare.

By 3 a.m. at home again, Fabulosa is madly vacuuming. "We just have to make sure the house is clean," she says.

"I think we should go to the hospital," I tell her. "Just to get situated."

The one-mile drive feels like a hundred. Contractions every two minutes. The side door to the hospital—the one we've always used—is locked. The overhead lights glare surreal. We wait and wait for a security guard to let us in, then walk and walk toward green elevators.

At the entrance to the hospital chapel, the Virgin Mary holds her giant crucified son. Not quite the image of motherhood I need right now.

Finally up in the maternity ward and a nurse tapes a hospital bracelet around my wrist. I already regret being here. Contractions come fast and deep and I lean over the birthing ball, try to remember the self-hypnosis from the CD. There's a switch you flip to turn the pain off, but I can't find it now. The room is too cold and too hot. I pull at the bracelet, claustrophobic. "Let's get the fuck out of here," I tell Fabulosa.

They've tried to make the maternity ward nice and homey, so it doesn't feel like a hospital, but it still feels institutional—it's like you're laboring in a Motel 8. The nurse says I'm six centimeters dilated. I'm crawling across the floor when she asks if I want the baby circumcised. I think maybe I've misunderstood, but I gather all focus of linear thought to answer her: "First of all," I manage, "*no*. And second... can't we talk about this kind of thing tomorrow?"

I feel like I'm on a bad acid trip. I'm walking down hallways, bright blur of doors and corners. Maybe I'm glad I wasn't so afraid, but now I feel like I've been lied to. It's not my fear or my bad attitude that's making this hurt. It just hurts.

Had Baby. Bring Coffee

Fabulosa's hand on my back helps and then doesn't help. I'm in a jacuzzi, but they want me to get out. Warm cold bright rest. They say I'm almost there, but they are lying. They don't know who I am. They don't know that I know about these things. I want to stay in the water. I'm falling asleep for odd moments between contractions. I'm sweating, shivering. "I'm scared," I admit. I'm standing in front of a sink, vomiting. I've only been here a couple of hours—it's just the beginning. *Fuck natural childbirth*. I want the drugs. I'm searching for the words to tell them. I am being led somewhere. The midwife is here. The room is dark. "Do you remember about pushing?" she wants to know. I do not remember. They are telling me to push with the contraction but I can't tell the difference between contraction and not-contraction. The midwife says I'm doing good, says it's almost over. I don't believe her, don't know why she's lying to me. My hip joint spasms and Fabulosa does something to make it hurt less. I am pushing, but I can't do it. He's too big. Or I'm not strong enough. Everything is dark. And I remember Giuditta on the CD promising that I'd stretch—no problem. It's cold in here. And what if I can't push him out? My timing is all wrong. What if they have to give me a c-section? Push now, they say. Good, they say. Then all at once the strange sound pain lights pull.

And Fabulosa cries soft gasp. And everything is empty.

Sudden as morning, he's on my chest. All pink and lung power. All fat and wet. Tiny fingers, berry mouth.

And they like him already. They *ooh* and they *aah*. They want to know what he weighs. The room is awash with light. "You didn't tear," the midwife says. "You stretched—no problem." It's only 7:16 a.m. And he weighs nine pounds eight. Number we should remember.

I ask Fabulosa for my cell phone so I can text Maia: HAD BABY. CALL WHEN YOU WAKE.

Baby Cosmo.

Maximilian Cosmo.

I text Uncle Donor: HAD BABY. BRING COFFEE.

12

Opening

Joan Labbe

I divulge the usual parts of my daughter's birth story as eagerly as the next mom, reaching for the promised land, that warm buzz of connection that comes from shared experience. Yet as I turn to leave, the smile so ready to arrive hardens and crumbles, proving itself a faulty structure. Why did I avoid those other parts of my story again, telling what is at best a half-truth? Why did I place one more stone in the dam holding back my torrent of secrets, creating an artificial, uncrossable divide between those other mothers and me?

I picture myself inching open the great gates, letting loose the rush of held back truth, and what I come up against is this: It would take too long. It would be too hard. It's way more than they realize they've asked. It's way, way more than they want to hear. And the one with the biggest ring of truth to it—my own fear. Fear of the spiraling, bottomless "I have no idea what to say to that" silence in which I would become lost. At home, after my kids fall asleep, and I'm left with me and the silence. Then I would drown in what I released. The fact I dared to free it would not save me.

Damned if I don't tell then, and yes, I'm pretty sure, damned if I do. Yet the desire to tell all of it, difficult, intimate, imposing as it is, remains. It will not be ignored or reasoned away.

So here it is. Picture a woman afraid of heights. She struggles for years with a therapist to inch off the ground. Relentless nightmares make her fear sleep. The constant challenge to her safety boundaries makes her feel the center of her self being stripped away. She spends an increasing amount of time curled up in a fetal position on her bed to make it to the next minute, then the next one after that. Her body gives her diarrhea and mysterious roving pains as she tries to pry her clinging, objecting, horrified feet off the ground.

Imagine this woman, after three years of grueling effort, getting to the point where she climbs a 40-foot rock wall. She looks down from the top. Body feels good. Fear is in check. Huge for her. Gargantuan. The reason she entered therapy. She will no longer live a life ruled by this fear.

Break out the champagne.

Then, because things now seem possible that never did when fear shrouded her in its veil every day, this woman awakens to the realization that something she's yearned for, but never considered she might be able to get, is at the top of Mount Everest. She's got to climb Mount Everest to attain what her reawakened desire, pushing her with the unbelievable force of being stuffed down so long, insists she have right now.

If you can picture the level of fear and disbelief climbing Mount Everest would raise in this woman, then you have a picture of what birthing my first child represented to me. Fear beyond fear. For ten years, I suffered from secondary vaginismus. Vaginismus is a psycho-sexual disorder in which a woman's vagina closes involuntarily. For some women, it is when a penis tries to enter. For me, it was any object. Secondary refers to the fact that I developed vaginismus after having intercourse, as opposed to finding myself with it the first time I attempted intercourse.

I believed my vagina was simply too small for anything to enter without pain. A lot of pain. Unendurable pain. Fear of that pain made me hot and dizzy if I so much as formed an intention to try to put anything in my vagina. When pressed by my therapist with the question, "Do you think you have a space in your vagina?", I answered, "No, not really. If there is one, it's really, really small." My therapist pointed out I previously had intercourse. How could my vagina be too small? I pointed out that if it was big enough, why did I develop this problem? I went through all the struggles of my agoraphobic counterpart while trying to put something, anything, the smallest thing that wouldn't disappear, in my vagina.

It wasn't lost on me that in order to get pregnant, sperm would have to get to my eggs. Once that miracle occurred, there would be internal prenatal exams. Then more internals in labor. Finally, something quite a bit larger than the pinkie finger it took me months to insert would have to fit through my vagina. The baby's head.

That huge, impossible head.

This impressive array of hurdles had for years caused me to file the idea of having a baby right beside "It would be nice to sprout wings, travel past light speed and fly to the planet Saturn someday" in my mind. After several years of therapy it was still tucked away there one evening when my therapist said oh so casually, in that exploratory way of hers, "You know Joan, you can get the smallest two dilators in your vagina comfortably. That means a turkey baster would fit. You could get pregnant if you wanted to."

That's all it took. One comment unleashed nine years of repressed longing, nine years during which, when friends asked my husband Sal and me if we were "trying," he inexplicably replied "yes" while I simultaneously said "no," causing them to wonder what that was all about. I wanted to be pregnant. Tomorrow. Sooner than tomorrow. All I could think about was babies and this new amazing notion my body could create one. The force of my longing shocked me. It thrilled me. It scared the daylights out of me. I sang with it. I cried with it. I curled up armadillo style with it. At times I hated my therapist for calling it up.

My desire to be pregnant was so overwhelming, it took a few months for things like exams and the actual birthing of the baby to enter my mind. Birthing felt like the larger problem. I had just recently held up the largest dilator to my therapist and asked, my face reflecting the clear insanity of the notion, "Can any woman really get this in her vagina?" Even with the promise of an epidural, the suspension of disbelief necessary to picture a baby's head coming through was far beyond my capacity.

Opening

The topic of episiotomy made me want to pass out. "Joan, you will seriously not care when you get to that point," my therapist insisted with all her "I've had two kids of my own" wisdom. How could I not care about my vagina being cut when my biggest fear is vaginal pain? My therapist didn't understand this problem after all.

"The part that hurts is your cervix opening," she told me the following week, "not your vagina." She wasn't fooling me. That baby had to get out of my vagina after it passed through my cervix and I wasn't buying her airy dismissal. If my vagina muscle could close involuntarily to keep things out, it could close involuntarily to keep a baby in. What would I do then, a massive episiotomy?

"Hey," I mused hopefully to my therapist another week later, "do you think if you told them it was psychologically necessary, you know, explained my history and stuff, they'd just schedule a c-section?"

"Well, that might work," she replied kindly.

Good enough. They could cut a hole in my stomach as long as nothing touched my vagina. Now there was only this pelvic exam problem. Deborah, my trusted Nurse Practitioner, had given me valium on my previous attempt. I sobbed from the moment my legs parted. Eager to prove I could get through an exam without valium or tears, I listened to my therapist's hypnotic tape, practiced religiously with a speculum, and sailed through my next attempt drug and trauma free. Deborah rewarded me with a basal body thermometer, some specimen cups, and a few plastic syringes as an improvement on the turkey baster idea.

Four months later, I threw myself into Deborah's arms as she held up my positive pregnancy test. My body, once so broken, was working.

After some early bleeding, I cried soundlessly through an internal ultrasound. Deborah's instructions specified an external one, but the technician insisted only an internal would tell us if my baby was alive at seven weeks. I cursed the idiot inventor of the probe for making it square for God's sake. It must have been a man. "The least he could have done was make it vibrate!" I insisted to my amused co-workers. Back home, I could not stop sobbing.

My almost-baby deserted the tomb of my body the following week. I went to bed for a long time.

Two months after my period returned, I was pregnant again. "Are you sure about your dates?" asked the ultrasound technician. I held up the chart showing the night I ovulated, proving my second baby was not growing.

I chose some pre-Everest warm-ups, infertility tests. Two were invasive. One shot dye through my tubes (Deborah held my hand and helped me breathe through that one). The second was an endometrial biopsy (I screamed and made Deborah promise never to do it again). In the midst of miscarrying, testing, and lighting candles for my lost babies, I exercised control over the only area I could. I figured out how to have orgasms, got that impossibly large dilator in my vagina, and had intercourse for the first time in ten years.

"Your vaginismus is resolved!" celebrated my therapist, presenting me with a backpack that folded up into a very small pouch. It represented my vagina opening. I tucked the backpack in a special place. Then I let her know how much her glee pissed me off. How could she smile and shop when here I was, unable to feel the happiness I had envisioned for years, cheated by my grief, my lost vision of the future, my lost, fleeting faith in my body?

Using progesterone supplements, I got pregnant a third time. Something different happened. This baby had a heartbeat. At 19 weeks, I found myself staring incomprehensibly at an ultrasound of something looking quite alive and babylike. Might this one stay alive and be born? Perhaps I should let go, just a teeny bit, of my need to believe otherwise and start thinking about how she (so the ultrasound said) was going to get out of my body.

Much had changed since I asked my therapist about the possibility of a scheduled c-section. Still, it felt huge to contemplate birthing again. I could endure exams. But I wanted a consistent person, someone to whom I wouldn't have to explain each time my need to put the speculum in myself and go slowly. I wanted a birthing environment that wouldn't feel scary and out of control, a place where I would be listened to, honored and supported.

My changing needs led me to a decision I couldn't have contemplated when I held up the largest dilator in disbelief. Forget the hospital with its succession of unfamiliar nurses and an OB I barely knew. I would plan a midwife-assisted birth at a nearby birthing center. Rotating appointments would acquaint me with four midwives, one of whom would be with me from the beginning of labor through the birth of my baby. The midwives would not perform unnecessary exams. They resisted interventions like episiotomies. The idea of laboring in a Jacuzzi tub felt decadent, and the words used by mothers who'd given birth at the birthplace mesmerized me. "Warm." "Safe." "Cared for." "In charge." "Comfortable." Even "empowered."

But there was no epidural there. As much as I now craved emotional security over drugs, what if I couldn't do it? I felt reassured by the fact that all I had to do was say the word and an ambulance would whisk me to the hospital two minutes away. The midwife would even go with me and stay till the baby was born.

I made the switch. Immediately, the midwives did shocking things. During visits, they sat down and made prolonged eye contact. My OB had hovered between the door and me, ready to check me off her long list. The midwives chatted. Yes, that was the only word for it. They remembered my name without glancing at a chart. The importance of my backup plan faded into a desire to avoid leaving this wonderful place.

Labor hurt. It hurt in ways you have to go through to know. Even the initial satisfaction I got fantasizing the demise of the birthplace nurse who'd clucked reassuringly at my fears, lowered her voice, and confided, "Labor is like bad cramps when you get your period. Nothing we women haven't felt before," faded swiftly in the face of the increasing intensity of the pain. It might have been my period for the first hour or two. Then it moved into a previously unexplored sphere. I focused on breathing techniques like a shipwreck survivor swimming toward the only object in sight. I focused to prevent my complete decline into panic.

I went into labor at midnight on a Friday while our cat chased a mouse around the TV and I insisted Sal let it be for heaven's sake. After 17 hours, I called the midwife, Jill. My contractions weren't close enough together consistently, but I was exhausted. "I'll meet you at the birthplace," she said.

I arrived covered in vomit and hopeful. I'd read about queasiness in labor. I yelped as Jill's fingers reached for my cervix.

"Yes, it's more intense in labor. Okay, you're not going to like this much. You're one centimeter." ONE CENTIMETER! "But the good news is you're 85 to 90 percent effaced."

This last bit of news did not replace the panic of 18 hours equals one centimeter. How long to get to the magic number of four to be admitted? Okay, first labors could be long. But when I did the math, this was ludicrous.

"I can't go through another night like last night," I managed to spit out past the large rock that had just taken up residence in my throat.

Only Jill's reassurance that "If you're not admitted tonight, I'll give you something so you can sleep" got me home. In the shower, my tears flowed with the water. One centimeter! After a few hours, Jill called. Sal's description persuaded her to have me come in again. One more whimpering pelvic check and a relief I can feel to this day washed over me. I was four centimeters. My body was working. I could settle in to the Jacuzzi and stay.

I fell asleep between each three-minute contraction, too exhausted to know I was drifting off, yanked back mercilessly each time by the heaving that forced me anew into its rhythm of pain. Then Jill started stretching me. "You have a narrow perineum," she informed me. "This will help".

The stretching burned horribly. If I could have described the searing pain I had feared so greatly yet never actually felt during my vaginismus, this would have fit the bill. The only thing that stopped me from begging for the epidural was the knowledge that to get it I'd have to get out of the water and put on clothes while enduring contractions. Ugh. I needed the water. I needed to not move. The idea of clothing was repulsive. Any kind of ride would be impossible.

"I can't do it. I can't do it. I can't do it," I kept saying. Yet for lack of a feasible alternative, I kept doing it.

About one a.m., I started to push. Too exhausted to stay in the tub, I tried the birthing stool. I tried being upright. I landed on the bed. I was thrilled. The hard part was over. On the birthing video, it never took more than three or four pushes for the baby to come shooting out. The pain of the last 25 hours was about to end, finally, blissfully. I would sleep forever.

Opening

"Can you see the head yet?" I asked after four pushes. Why was it taking so long? Jill gave me some tips on curling my chin and holding my breath. 40 minutes later, I had no energy left.

"How do you feel about an episiotomy?" asked Jill. "Do whatever you think is best," I mumbled. I did not care. My therapist was right. But I was also sure Jill's question meant my vagina was not capable of opening enough. That was why it was taking so long. My perineum was too narrow. This baby was not coming out.

"Joan, reach down and feel her head," Jill insisted, trying to re-energize me. With a mixture of resignation and curiosity, I reached down and felt my baby's head. It was amazing. There was so much hair on it. It was right there. Wow. Right there. Oh my God. It was stuck! Yes, this huge head was stuck there, just as I had feared, in my vagina.

Suddenly it came to me that this baby was exactly like that tampon I tried. I was so eager, so excited to be able to try one, I put it in when I was sure my period was about to start but before it actually started. It did not start. The tampon sucked me dry. It wouldn't come out. My therapist was heading to a meeting when I reached her. "Leave it in till I get back," she instructed. I hung up the phone. I realized it could not stay in. It was intolerable to have it in without my permission. So I yanked it, inch by painful inch, then a few huge violent tugs, OUT.

Except this baby was too big to yank out. So at 25 and ¾ hours, I started screaming. It was a noise unrelated to the pain of labor. In fact, it didn't seem related to my body.

"Joan, stop. Stop." Jill's voice was hard. The screaming miraculously ceased. "Joan, all you need to do now is open your legs wider. I've been telling you, but you're not doing it. Your baby doesn't have enough room to come through."

So this was it. After all my fears about pain, burning, being cut, my vagina closing, this was the part stopping me. This was what was left. I focused all I had on pushing my legs apart. They wobbled perhaps a half inch then retracted. It felt too open. Too exposed. It wasn't safe. Every instinct I had rebelled against opening. On the bed with the head of the baby I wanted more than life between my legs, I could find no room to negotiate with my fear.

So I did something else. "I can't do it," I gasped to Jill and Sal. "Please do it for me, please." Jill held one knee. Sal grabbed the other. I tucked my chin, held my breath the way I was supposed to for what felt like the first time, and pushed. The baby tore my uncut perineum and shot out between my held down legs. She was out. I had let them hold down my legs. I had not freaked out. It was done. She was here. It was done.

Jill was still there. "Push the placenta out," she insisted.

She reached for sutures. I had torn. Some places don't get really numb. My baby's face, alive, new, held me through the sewing.

Hands massaged my uterus, bringing back pain as if I was in labor again. Would Jill ever leave my body alone?

Not yet. I'd neglected to pee during labor. Now I couldn't, not even to the sound of running water, my savior after I had major surgery several years earlier and discovered I couldn't tolerate the nurse's attempt to catheterize me. The fact the opening in question was not my vagina had not helped. I couldn't open my legs for that hospital nurse. Even if my bladder burst.

But that was then. Now I gazed at a baby I'd believed would never arrive. Through ten years of vaginismus, a year of miscarriages, and half my pregnancy, I had barely let myself dream about her. She was here, breathing softly, mine. I'd endured 26 hours of labor, the stretching of my perineum. I'd let myself be forcibly exposed. That impossible head had burst through my too small vagina. I'd been sewn up. I could do this catheter thing. With my baby's face embracing my eyes and Sal's hand once again rendered bloodless by mine, I let one more fear go.

Shortly after I got home, I started to read a book by Penelope Leach. It began with an introductory section on childbirth. It's your baby's birth, her introduction insisted, not yours. I felt an unexpected anger at her words. Yes, it was my baby's birth experience. But it was also mine. I was born as a woman connected for the first time to her amazing, cavernous, stretchy-like-you-wouldn't-believe vagina that could tear and somehow heal. I was born as a woman with a body no longer broken. I was born as a woman on the other side of fears that had brought her to her knees over and over, but which never would again. I was born as a woman who

Opening

felt for the first time she lived not in a world of stop signs, but one of possibilities. I was born as the lucky caretaker of a little girl I named after my therapist.

I was also born that morning as a woman with a mile-wide-can't-figure-out-how-to-cross-it-and-it's-killing-me divide between the birth experience of almost every other childbearing woman and mine. Because although almost every woman wonders how something that large can come out of that space, their fear is not my fear. And we women talk about our child's entire birth yet somehow manage to avoid using the uncomfortable word "vagina." I was born into the secret clan of motherhood as the stepchild who causes embarrassment. I was born as a mother whose real birth story stops conversation.

So I offer it up here and wonder what may be born from the telling.

13

Granddaddy's Obstetrics

Frederica Mathewes-Green

My grandfather lived to be 94, and in many ways he was like a birch tree: small but springy and bright, with light filling his blue eyes. For over 60 years, he signed his name George Frederick Oetjen, M.D., and (although he told his daughters that "M.D." really stood for "My Daddy") being a doctor was the joy of his life. Many of those years he was an obstetrician, and once I had a chance to ask him about his obstetrical training.

There was a reason for my curiosity. I had just gone through my third "natural" birth, and I had been teaching the subject to pregnant women for years. But what did I really know about childbirth? Everything I believed was colored by a narrow range of experience: modern, middle-class, American birth practices. What had this experience been like for other women in other eras? What did my grandfather know that I didn't?

Of course, I had a sneaking suspicion of what his reply would be. I figured he'd say in a kindly tone, but with unmistakable condescension, that women are weak, birth-giving is dangerous, and the most important thing is to obey the wise (and presumably male) obstetrician. I expected one whose medical training began before World War I to be steeped in such thinking.

Was I wrong.

Grandaddy looked away, as if recalling a classroom of almost a century before. "I can remember my old professor of obstetrics," he said, "telling us about the Indians and how they would march along." *The what?* I thought.

Granddaddy's Obstetrics

He went on, "When an Indian woman went into labor she would step outside the line and give birth. After the baby was born the others would slow down, so she could catch up with them and go on. It was as easy as that. My professor told us that story, then said, 'If you men keep in mind that it's just a normal physiological event, and keep your hands off, and just let nature take its course, you'll get a normal baby and a normal delivery.' And I still believe it."

I was surprised to hear such "natural birth" sentiments being recalled from a Georgia classroom of 1917. While the story about Native American birth practice might indicate cultural naïveté, it indicated something else as well: a conviction that birth was an essentially healthy process. Far from relegating women to helpless passivity, or elevating obstetricians to god-like control, there was an expectation that women were strong and competent to give birth with minimal assistance.

Obviously there was a lot I didn't know about the obstetrics of the time. When I got a chance, I scanned his bookshelves until I found it: a red volume stamped in gold: "Obstetrics—Williams." *Williams Obstetrics* is still the standard textbook for obstetricians-in-training, though today's students enjoy a fresher version; my grandfather's was the 4th edition, published in 1917. Leafing through, I discovered aged sheets of paper slipped between the pages, containing notes he had made about obstetric cases under his care. One included the ominous words, "Puer Sepsis"—the dreaded "childbed fever" that claimed so many lives before sterile technique was fully understood. Another scrap of paper was headed "Final Exam" and listed numbered essay questions. It struck me that the questions could appear unchanged on an exam of today (for example, "What is your conduct of the third stage of normal labor?"), but the correct answers would be dramatically different.

As I read through the textbook I saw there gradually emerge a portrait of a very different time, and a very different approach to birthing. For example, today pregnant women are expected to go for early and regular prenatal exams. At the turn of the century, however, care consisted of monthly urinalysis and not much more. The woman would be physically examined only once, and even that one exam was not easy for the obstetrician to get, in that adamantly modest era.

J. Whitridge Williams wrote regarding prenatal care: "In private practice it is not necessary to examine the pregnant woman in the early months of pregnancy unless symptoms indicative of some abnormality occur...On the other hand, a careful and thorough examination is indispensable about six weeks before the expected date of confinement, and to neglect in this respect can be attributed the deaths of untold numbers of women and children. Usually this can be made much more conveniently with the patient in her own home and in bed than at the physician's office...Unless the physician fully appreciates the importance of this examination, and has learned to look upon the making of it as a bounden duty, he may sometimes be deterred by feeling that it is repugnant to the patient, and that she may object to it or even refuse it. My experience, however, has always been that a few words of kindly explanation soon smooth away all such difficulties...If, however, despite the exercise of the greatest tact on the part of the physician, and his insistence that such an examination is a necessity for her own sake, the patient persists in her refusal, the former has no alternative but to decline absolutely to attend the case."

As I continued reading, I discovered other ways the treatment of labor has changed. Many hospitals are cautious about letting women out of bed in labor; the attachment of fetal heart monitor and IV drip make this complicated, and epidural anesthesia makes it impossible. The toll may be in slowed labor; when the woman is allowed to move around as she likes, the process tends to pick up. 80 years ago, obstetricians were taught to let laboring women set their own pace: "During the first stage of labor the patient usually prefers to move about her room, and frequently is more comfortable when occupying a sitting position. During this period, therefore, she should not be compelled to take to her bed unless she feels so inclined."

The obstetrician's role in a birth like this was essentially that of a lifeguard, standing by in case of an emergency. Occasionally such a situation did arise, but transfer to a hospital was not a necessity, particularly for minor "operations" such as the use of forceps. Nevertheless, it's startling to imagine the settings in which our foremothers gave birth: "For the performance of an operation, it is advisable, even in private practice, to place the patient upon a narrow table. One that will answer the purpose quite satisfactorily is usually to be found in every kitchen, but, if a suitable table is not available, a satisfactory makeshift may be improvised by unscrewing the mirror from a bedroom bureau."

Much of my work as a childbirth educator had been aimed at helping women use natural pain-relief techniques to avoid medication. Medication for childbirth had been introduced with some controversy in the mid 19th century; some felt that it was contrary to Scripture ("In pain you shall bring forth children," Genesis 3:16) and others warned that only childbed pain induced a mother to love her child. Gradually anesthesia won acceptance, particularly after it was used by Queen Victoria. But the medications available then were of a very different kind from the epidural anesthesia available now.

"The most popular anesthetics are ether and chloroform," Dr. Williams wrote. "...Generally speaking, chloroform is preferable in normal labor, for by its use obstetrical anesthesia can be rapidly and safely produced. I believe that it is practically devoid of danger when properly administered, and should be used whenever there is time for its administration, unless the patient has conscientious objections to its employment." These must be those women who felt pain to be somehow necessary or redemptive. I and the women I taught didn't share that point of view, but just wanted to control and experience our births more fully by using drug-free methods to reduce pain.

As I taught my students, the worst pain of labor is late second stage, just before you begin to push. But it certainly won't look that way; it looks like the worst part comes later, at the moment of birthing the baby's head. For many women this is painless, or provokes an intense but brief burning sensation; it certainly isn't the time for anesthesia if you've avoided it so far.

Dr. Williams gave opposite instructions, however. "The choice of the time for its administration, however, is of great importance, nor should it be used before the latter part of the second stage, when the head becomes palpable through the perineum... When properly administered, the patient experiences marked relief after a few inhalations, but retains consciousness and is generally able to talk rationally. When the distention of the vulva is at its maximum, obstetrical anesthesia is not sufficient to abolish the pain, and it is my practice at that time to render the patient completely unconscious by increasing the dose of the drug."

At the time this edition of *Williams Obstetrics* was being written, feminists and social leaders like Mrs. John Jacob Astor were touting a new form of anesthesia called Twilight Sleep. This combined the previous method (ether or chloroform) with scopolamine, a drug that induced hallucinations and amnesia. It didn't reduce pain, necessarily, but it eliminated the memory of pain, and the memory of shameful exposure (at least the conscious memory of these; bizarre dreams and nightmares were not uncommon postpartum effects). After decades of widespread popularity, this artificial and purposeless drug cocktail was gradually rejected. Dr. Williams predicted as much decades before it reached its ascendance: "The method is not ideal, and it is my belief that it will gradually fall into desuetude, or at least that its use will be restricted to a small group of neurotic patients."

Should the doctor make an incision in the vagina to enlarge its circumference for birth? Natural-birth enthusiasts frown on routine episiotomy, believing that such an incision is not always necessary, and that natural tears are likely to be smaller than the one the doctor would inflict. Dr. Williams agrees: "Personally, I see no advantage in the procedure, as my experience is that ordinary perineal tears will heal almost uniformly if properly sutured and cared for."

The rate of cesarean delivery is cause for concern now as it was then. The female body is designed to give birth, and we all are descended from a long line of birthgiving women; the need for the radical intervention of cesarean section should be miniscule. Yet a fourth or more of births each year are cesarean, a figure caused by many factors including the litigious and malpractice suit-prone society we inhabit. Dr. Williams opposed the increasing reliance on the procedure: "There seems to be a growing tendency to regard cesarean section as the simplest means of coping with obstetric difficulties. At the present time I consider that the operation is being abused, and that not a few patients are sacrificed to the furor operativus of obstetricians and general surgeons who are ignorant of the fundamental principles of the obstetric art."

Granddaddy's Obstetrics

Of course, in 1917 cesarean delivery was still an extremely risky operation, due to the danger of deadly infection; Dr. Williams warned that ten percent of cesarean patients would die. He recommended alternatives that could be highly damaging, but were less likely to be fatal: forceps thrust high into the uterus, an incision through the cervix and lower uterine segment, reaching into the uterus to turn the child by hand, forcible dilation of the cervix, and cutting through the pubic bone.

Dr. Williams' opposition to unnecessary cesareans was matched with a belief the procedure should not be unnecessarily repeated; vaginal birth after cesarean was quite possible, even though there were some cases in which the previous incision had ruptured. "Certain authors consider it so real a danger that they have laid down the dictum, 'Once a cesarean, always a cesarean.' This is an exaggeration, as the accident is likely to occur only when the wound has been improperly sutured, or its healing has been complicated by infection."

I was surprised to see such a generally favorable approach to natural birth in a textbook from so long ago. But as I read on, the advice on caring for mother and child after the birth perplexed me.

Dr. Williams wrote: "It is a time-honored custom to allow the puerperal woman to sit up on the tenth day. This rule, however, should not be slavishly followed, and every patient should be kept in bed until the fundus of the uterus has disappeared behind the symphysis pubis. This frequently occurs by the tenth day, occasionally a day or so earlier, but very often not until some days later. Generally speaking, a two week's rest in bed is not excessive." As someone who had always been up and about the day after birth, it certainly sounded excessive to me.

Dr. Williams agreed with contemporary thinking regarding the high value of breastfeeding: "The ideal food for the newly born child is the milk of its mother, and, unless lactation be contra-indicated by some physical defect, it is the physician's duty to insist that every woman should at least attempt to suckle her child."

But the procedure he recommended sounded bizarre, to say the least. "Bathe the nipples with saturated boracic solution before and after each nursing...Until the milk appears, nurse three times a day, and don't give any other food unless otherwise directed." Dr. Williams went on to prescribe a regimen of military precision: "After the milk appears, let the child suckle, except after its bath, every three hours by the clock, from 6:00 or 7:00 a.m. to 10:00 or 11:00 p.m. Time one feeding so that it will come directly after the bath after which the child may be allowed to sleep as long as it will. Feed only once, or not at all, between bedtime and 6:00 or 7:00 a.m. As soon as the milk appears, write out a schedule for nursing and adhere to it, awakening the child at each feeding time if necessary. Before each nursing wash out the child's mouth with boric acid solution. After the first three weeks increase the intervals between feedings to four hours."

Regulating the child and insuring its compliance with the household schedule was apparently of utmost importance. "As soon as the child is taken from the breast it should be placed in bed and not disturbed. It should not be allowed to sleep at its mother's breast, nor should it be rocked or fondled after feeding. If these regulations be persisted in, the child will usually go to sleep within a few minutes after being put to bed, and if it wakens before the next feeding is due it will remain quiet. The importance of following these directions cannot be overestimated, for it is only by rigid adherence to such details that the child can be given regular habits, and its care prevented from becoming a strain upon all concerned."

Of course, the most taxing element of baby care is diaper changes, and Dr. Williams had no doubt that this could be regulated as well. "The physician should impress upon the mother and nurse the necessity of attempting to train the child to regular habits as to urination and defecation, and it is surprising how soon these may be formed if proper care is taken. For this purpose the napkins should be changed before each feeding, and after the first few weeks the child should be held over a small chamber at these times."

As I closed the bulky red volume, I felt that I had traveled to a strange time: a time when home birth was the norm, but home-birthing women were rendered unconscious at delivery: a time when breastfeeding was almost compulsory, but the infant was not allowed to sleep at its mother's breast; a time when doctors hesitated to do a hasty cesarean, sometimes preferring to saw through the woman's pubic bone. I went back to my grandfather with a question: as this training was seasoned by experience, how did he come to see the art of obstetrics? What was the most important part of assisting at the birth of a child?

"Patience and prayer," he said, "just remember that: patience and prayer. You can't rush childbirth; that's when you get into trouble. Just trust in nature to do a good job and don't interfere unless you're sure it's necessary."

He paused and looked off again, as if envisioning himself about to go in to deliver one more baby. "At old St. Luke's Hospital, there was a prayer framed over the scrub sink," he said, "and the last line of it always stayed with me. It read, 'For without Thy help we can do nothing.' It didn't say 'Without Thy help we can do a little bit'—it said 'nothing.' I always thought about that every time before I went in to a delivery. Young doctors today should just remember three things: you're there to help at an essentially normal process; keep your hands off; and keep praying—and you'll have a happy birth."

There didn't seem to be anything I could add to that but "Amen."

Postscript:

I was able to find the "MD Means My Daddy" poem on the internet. My mother used to quote this when I was little; apparently she really believed it as a child. It sounds early 20th century.

Whenever Daddy signs his name, he always writes M.D.,
So everyone will know that he belongs to me.
For M.D. means "My Daddy", or something just the same.
And that is why he always puts these letters in his name.
Some letters in his name are small, but these are not, you see.
He always makes them big like that because he's proud of me!

14

Blue Moon Baby

Erin Lassiter

My daughter was born five years ago on Super Bowl Sunday. She was headstrong then, and she's headstrong now.

The day started out with a baby shower. When I woke up in the morning, I felt rather blah, but I just chalked it up to the ninth-inning stretch. Clara was due in four days. It was all planned. I had a doctor, I was going to the hospital, and I was having an epidural. This birth would be by the American Medical Association book. Four years earlier, when my son had been born, I had opted for a birthing center and a mid-wife. Things had not gone well. My cervix had dilated to four centimeters after like what felt like ten years of labor, and then it had closed right back up again, seemingly unaware that it had not yet produced a baby. I ended up at a hospital screaming, half-naked, in a wheelchair, with a very smug doctor by my side whispering in my ear, "You really shouldn't be in that much pain." This time was going to be different. I had my compassionate female doctor, my ticket to a hospital bed, drugs prepped and ready to be fed into my veins. I was in control.

At the baby shower, I was freezing. Everyone was going about his or her business, tasting baby food and cutting cake, while I sat on the couch and shivered. I asked the hostess for a blanket and a thermometer. It appeared that I was running a fever so I called my doctor. On the way to the hospital, my father couldn't help but comment on how typical my behavior was: everyone had come to spend the day with me and I couldn't even be bothered to show them a good time.

Blue Moon Baby

At the hospital, I was diagnosed with dehydration. I could have sworn that it was labor, but machines don't lie. I was attended to by a lovely young intern who knew everything. She asked me intimate questions about my sex life in front of my father. The poor man didn't even know I was having sex. He was sure it was immaculate conception. I was discharged with the promise that I could come back when I was in labor.

The doctor had prescribed something for whatever I had and my partner took me to the pharmacy to pick it up. I felt my contractions getting stronger. I had to stop mid-step between each one. That was ten in the evening. By midnight, I was feeling the pain, so to speak. I called the hospital and my favorite intern answered. She told me that my contractions were too far apart to be considered real labor and that it was just the flu playing with my mind. She recommended Sudafed and asked for Scott, my partner. She told him that his job was to keep me calm, as it would probably be a few more days. Her famous last words to me were, "I know it hurts, sweetheart, but you need to save your strength for the real thing."

If I hadn't been raised with a morbid fear of authority, I might have told her to go get her gloves on because I was coming down to kick her ass. Instead, I drank the entire bottle of Sudafed, got down on my hands and knees, and went into a Buddhist trance. The pain became like nothing I had ever known before, but I didn't call out. I just clutched the bed and cried. The toilet became my new best friend. *If I could just go to the bathroom, I would be okay,* I kept telling myself. I forgot that it was a baby, not a bowel movement, that my body was working to expel.

Three o'clock in the morning rolled around. I called again. This time I got the nurse. She told me that she had talked to my friendly neighborhood sadist, the intern, and the bleeding was just residual from my exam earlier in the day. She didn't recommend that I come down to the hospital because I would just be sent right back home. The idea of going anywhere, much less having to make a round trip, seemed like a real bad idea. I got down on my hands and knees again. I'm not a particularly religious person but I prayed to God for strength. I tossed, I turned, I writhed, I clenched my fists, I moaned, but again, I didn't cry out. Words and sound seemed futile. It didn't matter what I said, no one could hear me.

At five o'clock in the morning, my water broke. I woke up Scott and said, "They have to take me now." He called the hospital. They suggested that he give me a shower because I surely had time. Meanwhile, alien forces had taken over my body. I was no longer in control of my functions. I had managed to avoid consciousness of the dreaded mucus plug during my first birth but there was no avoiding it this time. As I struggled to comprehend how I had given birth to a squid instead of a human, my body went to work and took what was left of my brain along for the ride. I convulsed with a contraction and lay down on the bed.

Another convulsion rocked my body to its core. I looked down and saw the top of a head between my legs. I said, "Scott, I'll take that shower later. She's crowning."

He responded with the wisdom of a rock. "Get it back up there!" he yelled.

Scott dialed 911 and got ready to deliver his daughter. Another contraction hit and little Clara came shooting into the world like a chicken on a June bug. She came like gangbusters, but she didn't cry and she was completely blue. I whispered, "Breathe, baby, just breathe, please baby breathe." I wiped what mucus I could with a towel and rubbed her back to keep her warm. My life flashed before my eyes as Scott received instructions from the 911 operator on how to cut the umbilical cord with a shoelace. For a few minutes, I thought we might lose her. As Scott struggled with the lace in one of my shoes, I filled with sheer terror. What if my baby died? How would I cope if she left me?

All of a sudden, the room began to fill with policemen, firefighters, and paramedics. They lined the walls around the bed. They filled the narrow hallway. Walkie-talkies buzzed and static voices spoke in code. Then everyone clapped. The room filled with the sounds of hands coming together in a cheer. I knew then that my little girl would be all right.

She was six pounds, 15 ounces. I saw it as a sign: my birthday is June 15th.

I hate to think to this day what I looked like at the time to all of those glorious people in the room. I lay naked on the bed with my insides poured out all around me. But I was floating. As I was wheeled down the driveway on a gurney, I noticed the moon. It was the second full moon of January. I had given birth to a blue moon baby and she had given birth to me.

Blue Moon Baby

I changed that morning in ways I might never have if I hadn't had to endure such an experience. I became aware of my own strength. So I made a pact with myself to teach my daughter to always trust her instincts and believe in her own wisdom. I never did kick the intern's ass. When she stitched me up, I could've kneed her in the jaw a couple of times, but I had gobs of Morphine running through my veins. Besides, my hardheaded little baby lay next to me loudly complaining about being poked and prodded and assessed.

You tell them! I thought. *Give 'em hell.*

15

First Memory

Georgia Tiffany

I do not remember being born. I cannot remember being anything before the herb garden, the one my father planted just below my bedroom window. Stone by stone, a deliberate piece by piece of a puzzle so carefully positioned in shape and fit, he almost did not need the mud to hold the stones in place, or the purple thyme to seam the stones. Perched on the back stoop, watching him, I stroked the fur of my black and white dog. I remember the organza summer dress tucked between my legs, the dress with tiny navy polka dots and the mini-pleated skirt that flared when I twirled, my arms out, head thrown back, eyes focused on the huge spinning bough of the pine. I remember the dizzy fall, the sharp pricks of needles on my legs, my dog barking. I remember the grass stain on my dress that my mother would never be able to wash out, and how my father condemned her for spending over two dollars on that dress, and then for permitting me to wear it outside to "play with the dog, for God's sake." I was four. I had words for all that. But I do not remember being born.

Every year, as a creative writing exercise, I ask my students, "What's the first thing in your life you remember?" I thought I believed, exceptions such as Helen Keller to the contrary, that we cannot remember what we have no language for. I'd wait for their eventual conclusion that language had to come before awareness could evolve into a "memory." I wasn't talking about photographs or stories relatives told that recreate a memory and someplace down the line we might assume we actually remember it ourselves. I was talking about real memory. And yet . . .

When anyone has asked about my first memory, I've recalled that back porch, my dog, the herb garden, the permanently stained dress. My father. And I've always thought I was four years old. But recently, when an ex-student asked me the same question, "What's your first memory, Georgia?", I saw myself sitting on the lap of Santa Claus, watching in horror as he removed his white beard, his pooched-out belly still shaking as jolly as the real Santa Claus, and he wasn't Santa Claus at all, but the man I called Uncle Max. Although I've had this memory before, the chronology hit me for the first time. I was four that Christmas of disillusionment. The incident on the back porch happened after Uncle Max moved to Utah. That summer couldn't have been my fourth summer. It had to have been when I was five, or thereabouts.

Suddenly all the memories, and their chronologies, become "or thereabouts," and my dissolving ability to pinpoint time prompts another question: Can we remember nothing but what we're capable of confronting or willing to reveal, if only to ourselves?

I saw the headline in a local paper dated December 1, 2004: *Netherlands hospital carrying out euthanasia for a few terminally ill babies.* The reporter documented several such mercy killings in 2003, Vatican outrage, and a list of the hospital's qualifying examples such as extremely premature births, epidermosis bulosa—a rare blistering disease—and severe cases of spina bifida—cleft spine: incomplete closure in the spinal column resulting in neural tube defect.

And then I remembered March 17th, four days after my third birthday: the peach chenille bedspread, fragrant as newly laundered sheets dried in the winter sun, my mother lying on her side. Me curled up close with my head next to her bent arm that rests on the pillow. The whole bedroom smells like my mother—a warm soapy smell—and the sheets full of cold and light, and she's going away soon. When she comes back, she tells me, she'll bring me a new doll. Or at least that's what I remember her saying. *I remember.* The smells, the dim light under the ivory shade of a small crystal lamp beside the bed, my mother's face, my one hand reaching up to touch her cheek when she says she will go away, my other hand exploring the texture of that chenille bedspread, stroking and fisting the raised furry part with my fingers.

Were words like crystal, ivory, chenille already accumulating in my head that enabled me to recall this? No photographs record that moment. I'm convinced no one told me this memory. But the sensory images must have been stored just waiting for language, and the article summoned those images. My first memory. Not when I was four, but when I was barely three. The smell of my mother. The touch of chenille. My breath accumulating on a window of waiting. How much farther back might the memory go?

The night my mother left, it snowed. I did not know she had gone until morning when I sleepily pushed open the door of my parents' bedroom. Snow-dusted branches of the maples curtained my view through the living room window where I stood to watch all day for my mother to return, and the next, and the next. How many days, I don't know, and when I ask her, she says she does not remember.

The questions are old ones: Does it take language to remember? Are there other processes inside us that both store and access what we call memory?

My mother came back without the new doll, but I'd missed her so much, I didn't care. Do I remember seeing the old white Ford turn into the driveway, my father taking out her suitcase from the back seat on his side of the car, then walking around to open her door? Did I have words for my mother then, the way she slowly negotiated one leg, then the other, from the car to the ground and stood tentatively—pale, fragile, sad? Did she see me so happy and waving?

The doctor assured my mother that it would be best not to name him, not to see him, that he could never survive in the world. My father concurred. Insisted. The doctor, I'm told, had projected my mother's baby to have an expected life span of five days.

Without a name, my brother stayed alive 45 days in the hospital. How did my mother go to sleep each of those 45 nights knowing that? Sacred Heart Hospital.

110

First Memory

Less than a mile from our house. My mother has saved the hospital receipt in her dark oak memory box. The total bill: $91.50.

Baby Boy Tiffany. Born March 18th, 1945. My brother.

I want to believe he remembered for his short life the sound of night snow sifting off the pines that shadowed the dimly lit parking lot of the hospital, dots of ice gently ticking, some adhering to the windowpane. I want to believe he could see from his miniature bed the heavy frost on the glass that morning of the 24th just before the weather cleared. I want to believe there is some beauty stored in his memory of being alive on this earth. But then must he also remember hosting the deformed spine, carrying it into the world? And must my mother always remember the distorted body that grew inside her?

"Spina bifida?" I ask her.

"I don't know," she says. "It sounds familiar."

16

Estrangement/Arrangement

Carmen Gimenez Smith

My husband is unwilling to guess when I'll go into labor but it's all I do. I want to receive an appointment card in the mail with a kitten hanging off a tree branch. There's a dialogue bubble above his head that says, "Hangin' In There." On the other side it says:

> You will be giving birth on April 1, 2006 at 4:55 p.m.
>
> Please call to reschedule at least 24 hours
>
> before your scheduled appointment.

The home stretch, the last lap, the third trimester. Her due date falls right in the center of the semester. Someone phones in a bomb threat to the university where I teach so class gets cancelled. Thank you, bomb threatener, for the extra day with my feet up.

These days, I feel I'm owed something. I'd like to belong to the culture that showers sweets and adulation on pregnant women.

I write little notes here and there for this book. In a few weeks, I'll be typing with a baby cradled in the crook of one arm, her eyes twitching in dream.

There is barely room for me in my body. My daughter is unquiet. I like the feeling of lying on my back because the books say not to and because it stirs her up.

The tumor in my mother's head was formed in her like I was once formed. Cells after cells duplicated into interloper. It's in its own sac, the thing in her head. Her doctor says it should come out within the year. The life of a baby.

Estrangement/Arrangement

She'll be fine, I repeat as mantra. It's me, after all, protecting my daughter from my mother's illness. I push it away from us both. I wish for the brain to absorb it like a fetus absorbs the homunculus.

When I was very small I imagined I lived in a crib in a red bedroom inside of my mother's body.

My mother's body could hardly keep me. Her body and mine were incompatible so that her body attacked mine with antibodies. I was born to transfusions and tubes. Yellow and livid. She says she prayed so hard her eyes hurt.

For two weeks, prodromal labor. *Precursory, or preemptive,* suggests Kamy, my midwife, although that possibility fades on the third day. Prodromal, sometimes cruelly called false. One night I shuffle up and down my hallway wrapped in my robe and in a blanket, shuddering and shivering. This labor is nothing like I thought it would be, like it was promised by all the well-wishers who suggest the second one is always easier.

The prodromal labor is the first lesson my daughter teaches me. What we will do together for the rest of our lives, solve each other's problems around time.

My mother recedes although I talk to her every day. *Now that I know,* she tells me, *I feel better.* I dart in and out of her world.

Meanwhile, my son grows charming. He likes to say *Mama, joke* when something funny happens. *Mama, ache-ache?* he asks with feigned sincerity when I am writhing in the bed. When he was born, I decided he wouldn't see me cry and in the last few days, that idea has gone out the window and he soothes me using the words I use to soothe him. *Sokay, Mama. Sokay.*

Mama, hold you. Mama, cuddle. Mama, work? Mama, fix it. Mama, clean it.

He talks to his sister through my skin. He wants her to come so that they can play. He thinks she will come fully formed.

Nights, I watch him from the inside of my pain which gives everything a hollow tin sound. Our routine is built around the pain. We eat a lot of take out. I slip into my bathrobe and wrap myself in the blanket to say, *This is beginning.*

Since it didn't start the last time, it might mean to start this time.

Pain as message. Pain as practice. Pain as matter. Every prodromal night, I tell myself that I am bigger than the pain. Platitudes about pain I read in books. I am scholarly about pain. Generous with it. Surrender my body to it.

I pace the hallway because I remember that laboring women pace. The dog walks underfoot.

One day the pain is so bad I can barely stand it. It feels like useless pain. I understand that it's useless and that my baby won't be born from it and then the pain gets so bad I call Kamy who tells me to go to the hospital.

They put me into a hospital bed; the mattress is as thin as a slice of bread. Do I call my mother?

A nurse straps me to a machine that measures my contractions. I'm in prelabor because of pain. My other midwife, my friend Tawnya, arrives. She begins by telling me about her drive over while she assesses the situation, my pulse, the printout from the machine she explains. There's the articulation of my decision to homebirth: the hospital's rude machine and my tattooed midwife counting my contractions with her head while telling me about her belly dancing class.

They tell me I need to rest and give me something for the pain. They tell me to come back if it starts again. My husband and Tawnya hustle me out of the hospital like it's a bad party. To tell my mother, to not tell her. I want to protect her from the anxiety I felt for a few moments: I might lose this baby.

But I need her.

My mother and I make light of it on the telephone—what we know to do with trouble. I tell her about the uncomfortable bed, the cold room and she tells me different stories about being in the hospital. Hearing the storm of diarrhea in the bed next to her when she was in labor with me. She wondered, *Who could be doing that? What do they look like?*

We stamp down both our crying and offer each other our happy voices like that O. Henry story in which the couple sells their treasures to buy each other a gift which is meant to embellish their treasures.

The hospital question looms over the conversations. Maybe it's a remedy to her story. Her anxiety is a charm against anything bad happening.

She calls me over and over.

Estrangement/Arrangement

She tells me the stories of her pain so I have context.

And then suddenly like a quick and violent storm the pains pass and I am back to being just pregnant, on the cusp of labor. The calendar suggests I am still at least 11 days from having this girl. She plans to stay for the entirety of her term, perhaps longer.

She tells me she plans on staying in that terrifying adolescent voice I have created for her. The one she uses to tell me she's pregnant, that she hates me. The one that she uses to tell me, *I wish I was never born.*

Languid malaise overtakes me but I don't call it that because of the *mal,* the something bad it suggests. Pregnancy makes me superstitious; I'll believe in anything. My husband indulges my naps and my insistence that he changes our son's every diaper.

On the day before she is born, I attend a student's thesis committee. My belly is bullet shaped. We talk about arrangement. Estrangement. Derangement.

My colleague and friend Connie, pregnant too. We are two more in the room.

I think I'm talking like I'm not pregnant. The non-mother, the professor with the slender belly.

That night. Am I prodromal again? I crawl about the floor. *Call the midwives,* I tell my husband. He says, *We have plenty of time.*

My body is a transition. All our progress is an unfolding.

I sit on the toilet but imagine myself sleeping in the bed. This girl doesn't know her body. Mother as estrangement.

I crawl around the floor while my husband is in bed. My histrionics shame me. I want to be that good birthing mother who has an orgasm. *Please,* I say. *Check me,* I ask. He learned the first time around how to measure a woman's cervix. *Cockwife,* I call him.

It's different, he says, his fingers in my body. My son sleeps quietly near this examination. The light in our house diffuses the moment. The dog's collar clicks against the floor where I rest my head. I listen for the coming train. Mother as derangement.

These are my last moments like Death Row. Where's my last meal, where's my tranquilizer? Dead Mother Walking. I assess what's around me, the shape of the room, the light in the bathroom, my son's repose in our bed.

My mind wanders, altered by fear and boredom and pain. How must my mother's head feel? That I spend time thinking about her tumor in terms of fetal development, that it's a living changing thing so will it be born tonight too?

My husband calls and the midwives come. In the interim, I fold laundry on the floor in anticipation of guests, pause for contractions. Mother as arrangement.

I am disappointed for these reasons: no birthing pool. Where's my Boards of Canada CD? I am thrilled for these reasons: My son sleeps. It's almost over.

I say, *Call Barry,* my father-in-law, as to not have the bother of worry over my son, the thing I most fear.

Five minutes after, the midwives, Kamy, Tawnya and Mel arrive. A moment after they've put a chuck pad under me, I feel a pop in my stomach. I think, *She's dead*, but it's only my water breaking.

I think she's dead, so what would that have meant? *Do I still have to push this baby out?*

Then the thrum of her heartbeat. Like gulps of water. That sound.

The endless pulse of the pregnant body. The circular time of my body, my mother's, my daughter's and so on.

I say, *Put on the Brad Mehldau,* or any music that might reach inside me and calm the bothered nerves in my body. A laserlike curing hum. As a child, I suffered terrible stomach aches and my mother would rub my belly and hum rhythmically. I want that.

I want my mother there too but not her terror. I'll shield her from my pain. From seeing any suffering, even this kind. Estrangement.

I won't be pregnant anymore and that is where the emptiness begins.

My mother hovers over my labor even when she's not in the room.

Time pushes me rudely through the works of pain.

Estrangement/Arrangement

I am afraid to push. Because of the last time. Because of how bullied I felt by my body. *Do I have to push?* I ask. Tawnya is a friend so I feel less interested in appearing proficient at this, how a doctor might have made me feel. She has witnessed much of my ineptitude at other things.

I summon up the eighth grade race in which I ran the mile and how it became painful and how I managed, because of shame, to keep running. I was ashamed because I never went to practice, wasn't really a runner.

No, your body knows what to do, she answers. She rubs my feet. This is— because of all the erotic energy in the room from my body and the reaching, sweating, pulling, the smells—like an orgy.

Time and its tethers loosened from me, me from them.

My husband squats behind me. Holds my body up. *Figuratively and literally.*

In between contractions is like in between takes in a film. We joke, our shoulders relax. We tease Kamy who sits in the hallway with the stomach flu.

I won't push. Because of the last time.

Passive descent. My body forces her out. My mind does nothing.

Descent. Decent, distant moving away. I try to move up out of the moment with my head. Against hers.

I push and know the shapeliness of her body. Push again and feel my daughter crown then sneak back into my body. *One step forward two steps back.*

I push and through that pushing. Crying. Ugly as a welterweight, she emerges. No one is ready for her and for this, I am proud. That I was efficient. Proficient.

A story from my mother: When I was born, the nurse wheeled me in to the room from the nursery in one of those clear bins. I was wrapped in a pink blanket and my mother was still disappointed about not being able to name me Natasha. My father would choose my name.

Then it occurred to her. This I have to take home. For good.

In the body, a baby is safe and conceptual.

When she tells that story, it's about terror although she doesn't say so, which is why we laugh. *How can it be about terror?* she laughs ironically.

We've both been bound in terror these months.

117

Being born has battered my daughter, an inverted triangle on her forehead where she passed the birth canal. Her nose is tilted right. Already thinking of her beauty because I know she might need it.

She's covered in blood and vernix and mucus. Her first coat. For weeks, we still pick vernix off her body, unwilling to give her a bath.

Her mewing is nothing like her brother's and this is the first shock.

My body is spent and still I take her.

I do want to hold my son for one last time. I didn't know that all that would be all over so soon. But he is sleeping with my father-in-law in the other room. He doesn't know how this house has changed.

Someone helps me up and I wobble like a fawn. *Who has the baby?* The house buzzes inside my ears. Someone puts a blanket over my shoulder. It's my Sesame Street blanket from childhood.

In the shower, afterpains, bleeding. The thud of adrenalin in my heart. If I could have stood there longer to hide from my daughter.

Then again, it was a hollow in me that she wasn't there. Absence so that I didn't dry off before she was in my arms, trembling. My love is split in two, one for each child.

When I hold her.

When she is against my body, eating me alive.

My daughter fits me like a key. She's my book.

17

Don't Even Bother:
The Case Against Childbirth Preparation

Kelley Cunningham

Do you feel that you were well prepared for childbirth? Were you able to distinguish the mucous plug from snot as you peered into the john for signs that labor was starting? Did you do your kegels while riding the subway to work, quite amazed that you could be doing something so intimate in such a public place while everyone around you was unaware? Did you pack a tennis ball in your hospital suitcase so your partner could rub your back with it, like I did for my first baby?

I'm betting that you had other ideas about what your partner could do with that tennis ball once the real pain hit.

Let's face it: childbirth preparation classes are a whole lot of hooey. Maybe we expect too much of them, because nothing can prepare you for the moment of ghastly realization that this kid is coming out and it's going to hurt like nothing ever has. And that you can't go home, have a glass of wine, and forget the whole stupid idea. All the tidbits of advice they give you fly out the window, the first being the flipping tennis ball. It won't hurt to play the Enya CD, mama, but it certainly won't help.

My decidedly un-P.C. picture of childbirth preparation classes may seem harsh to glowing and clueless moms-to-be. But the truth is that they only offer them to give you something to do now that your feet have become too swollen for shoe shopping. What else is there to do now that you've ordered the crib and laundered all the newborn onesies in Dreft?

Back me up, all you experienced moms out there. Did you really bond more closely in the class with your husband as he sat behind you, legs akimbo? How oddly voyeuristic was it to watch all the other couples doing this? I sure as heck didn't want to go out for a romantic dinner afterwards. I just wanted to go home and try to forget the sight of the woman next to me splitting her maternity leggings while she panted. The only conceivable (pardon the pun) purpose I can think of to this experience is to give you an idea of how many people are going to be looking up your yanni when you're spread-eagled on the table.

Did your Lamaze instructor tell you to pinch your husband's hand progressively harder while he panted so he could feel how a contraction feels? What a helpful exercise! That's like trying to explain how a guillotine feels by giving somebody a haircut. Look, I'll never know what it feels like to get slammed in the nuts, and there's no way he will ever remotely understand what childbirth feels like.

I love my husband and God knows the poor guy tried his best as a labor coach, but maybe, just maybe, he didn't belong in the delivery room. He was way out of his league. (Hell, I was way out of my league!) Perhaps we should at least give men the option to opt out. I wouldn't blame them. God knows I would rather have been chain-smoking in the waiting room than sweating in the delivery room if I had had the choice.

Childbirth has been women's work since time immemorial and perhaps that's the way it was meant to be. I suppose I'm glad my husband could see his children being born but this is a man who nearly passed out the first time because he forgot to eat for 12 hours. The second time he also forgot to eat and almost passed out when the OB asked him to cut the cord. The nurse had to help him into a chair while I'm pleading, "Hey…a little help here! I'm in a bit of pain!" The third time he wisely got an EggMcMuffin and munched it while his third son came into the world. This is absolutely true, I swear. All the while chatting with my OB about going out for martinis. I think the thing that fascinated him most was the contraction ticker-tape machine. He would kindly inform me that another one was coming up and boy oh boy it looks big!

I think the only thing more annoying would be a man who is way TOO involved. You know the type who says, "We're pregnant!" No, ding dong, your wife is pregnant. Put away the camcorder and get her some ice chips, stat.

There was something romantic about the old days with the smoke-filled waiting rooms and the pacing fathers. The nurse throws open the swinging doors and says, "Mr. Cousineau, you have a healthy son!" And he passes out anyway just like Ricky Ricardo but at least I don't have to deal with it. Then he gets to hand out cigars and get slapped on the back by all the other expectant fathers. Men need that bonding and they can't have it now that they're holding our knees next to our ears while we push.

I'm kind of like an animal when I'm sick or in pain. I want to be alone. Just let me crawl behind the sofa to die alone, thank you. Don't tell me how great I'm doing.

Like all earnest first-time moms, when I discovered I was pregnant I couldn't wait for the Lamaze classes to begin. I was planning on a natural delivery. No drugs for me. I can take pain!

I once ran a ten-mile road race with temperatures in the single digits. Thanks to a sadistic dentist, I had a root canal with insufficient novocaine. I pierced my own ears after a few beers. I skied in minus-15-degree weather until my nose was frostbitten. I drank a frat boy under the table in a shot contest. I am total chick macho. I can run with wolves. Women have been giving birth for millions of years and I can too!

Well, after pride cometh a fall, otherwise known as pitocin. They cranked up the IV and I had a contraction that tore me in two. I thought for sure someone had disemboweled me but the nurse looked at the monitor, merely shrugged and said, "Oh, that was a good one." At that point, I knew the only way Enya would help is if she were the one having the baby instead of me.

When I started to panic and became convinced that I could not possibly climb this Everest in front to me, the nurses reminded me of all the helpful tips I learned in childbirth preparation class.

"Don't work against your body. Work WITH your body. Just go with it."

All I know is that this body I'm unfortunately inhabiting at the moment is in a bit of a quandary from trying to pass an ICBM missile through an opening which God in his infinite wisdom made absurdly inadequate for the purpose. Therefore, I am reacting with grimaces of pain contorting my face.

"It's good pain. It's pain with a purpose!"

Come over here so I can punch you in the jaw. That's pain with a purpose too.

"Take three quick breaths, then hold it and push!"

Push what?

"Don't grunt like that. You'll have a sore throat in the morning."

I'll be dead in the morning if there's a God in heaven.

"Channel that womb energy."

Huh?

I knew then that even the nurses thought it was all bullshit, but what else can they say? They have to talk you down off the ledge somehow. If they said, *"Lady, you're on your own. Believe it or not, you'll get through this like everyone else,"* it wouldn't be very helpful. But at least it would be honest.

Maybe we should take Prissy's advice. In *Gone With the Wind,* she wanted to put a knife under Melanie's bed to cut the pain in two. Why the hell not? It's as good an idea as any other.

Every mother remembers her babies' births until her last breath. I won't go into details about the nauseating narcotic haze, or waiting for the anesthesiologist to stop by after his coffee and gossip break to administer epidurals that didn't take or worked too well. The forceps. The episiotomies. The hemorrhaging. All I know is I got shit karma in the Wonderful Childbirth Experience department.

Whenever I relate my birth stories to Earthy-Crunchy Moms, they're convinced it was the episiotomy that made everything go south for me. They tell me if I had massaged my moonachie with organic cocoa butter, an episiotomy would not have been necessary. Then I mention that my baby was nine pounds seven and they slink away, horrified. No one's hoo-hah is that big and I daresay that even a Costco sized vat of cocoa butter wouldn't have done the trick. Anyway,

Don't Even Bother: The Case Against Childbirth Preparation

I wanted that baby out of me so badly I would not have cared if they sawed me in two to hasten the process.

Another admission that will further sully my chances of winning Mother of the Year is this: when the baby was finally born, I didn't cry with joy. I didn't yearn to hold him. I merely looked up to see if he was breathing and let my head fall back onto the bed. I was so utterly relieved that the agony was over that that's all I could think about. Oh, after a few moments, I started to get curious about the tiny slimy creature pooping on the french-fry warming tray, but only after it sunk in that I wasn't going to die.

Thank God we came through it. By some monumental lapse of reason, I returned to the Maternity Pavilion twice more. I've got three wonderful sons, spider veins, and a little stress incontinence to show for it all. Happy ending.

But when I hear about women who had un-medicated births in hot tubs, or how for them pushing wasn't anything like the excruciating hell I experienced, I start to twitch. *"It was such a relief to push!" "My focal point was a picture of my husband on the wall and before I knew it she was born!" "My Doula rubbed my back with dong quai, did a hula dance, and fed me raspberry tea. It took all the pain away!"*

Well, I don't buy it for a minute. You are so full of shit. I don't like you, I don't trust you, and my kid is not going to play with your kids, you evil, Stepford-wife pods! Don't make me beat you about the head with this brand-new Baby Bjorn.

Every few weeks there's another baby that just pops out in the cab on the way to the hospital. I love the stories of the women who go to the ER with a case of indigestion that turns out to be full-term twins. I have to say I just don't get it. It is absolutely incomprehensible to me.

Strangely, some of the women I know who have had the easiest labors are the biggest wusses with anything else. They couldn't run a block without getting winded but they breeze through labor without so much as a twinge.

God knows what I did in a past life that earned me the honor of being the Rotten Childbirth Poster Child in this one. Wait, I know. I was a childless Lamaze instructor. That's gotta be it.

18

Another Day, Another Blessing

Diana M. Raab

In the latter part of my teen years, my nights were obsessed with recurrent nightmares about never being able to bear children. I would wake up in the middle of the night in a cold sweat and have to run to the bathroom to take a shower. During those nightmares, my babies were lost in different places—shopping centers, bathrooms, while sleeping. In reality, I only had one miscarriage at the age of 27, but the road to having three healthy children was surely a rocky one.

Almost immediately after graduating university, I landed an irresistible job as Director of Nursing in a chronic care hospital. At the same time, my husband Simon stepped into the business world to open an innovative engineering company.

We had worked for five years before entertaining the idea of raising a family. Even though our professional worlds rolled with excitement, at the age of 27, I knew that my ability to conceive was quickly slipping away. One evening during a candlelight dinner in our one-bedroom apartment in downtown Montreal, we both agreed it was time. Within a few months, we happily received a positive pregnancy test.

Simon and I bubbled with enthusiasm, and like most inexperienced mothers-to-be, I saw no harm in broadcasting the news, making down payments on baby furniture, and eating for two. Within the first six weeks, I donned maternity clothes and received congratulatory phone calls from friends and relatives from around the world. At ten weeks, I began bleeding.

As luck would have it, the mishap occurred on the weekend when my obstetrician, Dr. Mok, was out-of-town. At two o'clock in the morning, I was ripped out of bed with some serious cramping and bleeding. In the hope that it would pass, I laid back down for a few more hours, petrified to move. When the bleeding became worse, we decided it was time to head out to the local emergency room department. Two hours and three doctors later, the attending physician entered my curtained-cubicle and told me I could get dressed and go home.

"I'm giving you a prescription for a medication to stop your contractions," he said. "Take one tonight and then call your doctor on Monday morning."

After a restless weekend, I phoned Dr. Mok. "I cannot believe it," he said. "Your ultrasound on Friday was perfect. We heard the baby's heartbeat and saw your baby move."

On that Friday, Simon and I had left his office, glowing and with the sound of the baby's heart echoing in our ears. Never before had I ever felt such elation— the bliss of bringing a new soul into the world, a baby who began as the seed of love between Simon and myself.

Dr. Mok suggested for us to wait and see. "I don't want to jump to any conclusions. For now, just stay at home for a few days, and please don't do anything crazy."

Three days later while preparing a steak dinner, I began cramping once again; this time, the cramps were much stronger than those on the weekend. I ran to the bathroom. I knew that it was the end; my nightmare was coming true. We phoned Dr. Mok who met us in the emergency room. Within an hour, the nurses rolled me into the operating room for a dilation and curettage. After the procedure, I remained in the hospital for two more days. The emotional pain seemed deeper than ever imaginable. I cried uncontrollably and when least expected. Simon's kisses and hugs barely consoled me. How could women survive such a horrific event alone?

It took me a very long time to accept our loss. It was particularly painful being in close proximity to other pregnant women or even catching a glimpse of babies. Back then, we lived in a small apartment across the street from a park, which was frequented by women pushing baby carriages. On some days, I had to draw my curtains closed tight, because the sight and sounds of babies sent me dripping with grief. All the visuals were a painful reminder of my failure.

After six months of unprotected relations, the chances of another positive pregnancy test looked grim. Dr. Mok suggested another dilation and curettage, just in case remnants of the miscarriage were preventing me from getting pregnant. He also recommended marking my morning temperatures on a graph to detect my ovulation cycle. At the same time, Simon's sperm count was evaluated and those tests indicated that the problem was with me. Because my miscarriage was so unexpected, Dr. Mok decided to investigate even further.

He ordered for me to have a test called a *hysterosalpingogram* to detect the status of my reproductive system. This test, done in the radiology department, uses contrast dye injected into the uterus through the vagina and cervix. The uterine cavity fills with dye so the radiologist can detect any blockages.

From the waiting room, the older solemn radiology nurse called me into a small dark room with no windows and asked me to change into a hospital gown. She closed the door. In my puke green gown, I sat at the edge of the table waiting for the radiologist to enter. I glanced around the cold walls, which offered no solace. While waiting, I wondered if the one time I swallowed an LSD pill as a teenager in the sixties could have resulted in all this. After all, my mother never had difficulties getting pregnant and these things were supposedly inherited. Finally, a young radiologist entered, shook my hand, and smiled as he adjusted the computer screen. I tried to channel my way into his thoughts, to no avail.

"Today we'll be doing a *hysterosalpingogram*. If there is an obstruction, we'll spot it right away," he said robotically, nudging his chair closer to the computer.

I lay down on the table and he said he'd be inserting the dye. After moments of silence, he turned to me with his pen pointing to the computer screen and said, "What you have here is a double uterus, otherwise known as a *bicornate uterus*. As you can see, your uterus is heart-shaped with a septum in the middle, splitting it into two parts. The reason you miscarried was because your baby implanted itself in the left side, and my thought is that it didn't have enough room to grow

126

there. This condition is also associated with an *incompetent cervix*, which is more common than a double uterus." I knew that this meant that my cervical muscles were too weak to remain closed.

The diagnosis of incompetent cervix is usually made during the second trimester when a pregnancy is suddenly lost. The only way to carry a baby until term is by having something called a *McDonald* or *Shirodkar Technique*, a fancy name for a surgical suture placed around the cervix, done in the hospital under general anesthesia.

After my *hysterosalpingogram*, Dr. Mok suggested a consult with a surgeon for a second opinion—an unforgettable appointment. The surgeon's office was in the dark and dreary hospital basement, situated right next to the morgue! That in itself was not very encouraging and I swore the surgeon looked as if he could be a mortician. He coldly concluded that, in addition to having a cervical suture, the only way to carry a baby to term was to have a risky, major surgery to unite both my uteri.

"Otherwise," he said, "your baby will never have enough room to grow."

I implored him to suggest the most conservative treatment for my problem.

"If you were my wife, I would suggest the surgery."

There was something creepy and untrustworthy about this guy. His greased-back hair, dirty finger nails and lackadaisical demeanor made me feel ill-at-ease. Simon and I reluctantly thanked him and drove home. The following day we made an appointment with another surgeon. Much to my chagrin, he also recommended surgery.

We marched into Dr. Mok's office to share the news from the two consults. We waited only for a few moments in his tidy waiting room decorated with contemporary Chinese décor. A big coffee table in the center was splattered with baby magazines—another reminder of my failure. Why didn't they have golf or infertility magazines? The nurse welcomed me back and directed us to the two chairs facing Dr. Mok's desk. Behind his desk were poster-size glamour shots of his three children. On the credenza below were group pictures of his family. Part of me was inspired by the photos, and another part was immensely jealous.

Something about Dr. Mok instilled both of us with confidence. He was a good-looking middle-aged Chinese obstetrician in his mid-forties with a busy practice who had enough experience and enthusiasm for his work. He seemed like the type of person who would do anything to help us have children. We wanted to trust him with this task.

He pushed the tear-drop wire-framed glasses higher up on his nose.

"You're a nurse, so I know you'll understand what I'm about to tell you. An incompetent cervix is easy to treat. However, a *bicornate uterus* presents a different set of issues and complications. My thought on this is that as long as you've got patience, you can have babies. I'm willing to work with you so that surgery won't be necessary, but you must promise me one thing—not to lose hope. You *will* have children."

Simon and I looked at one another and nodded. My eyes bloated with tears. Dr. Mok had told us just what we wanted to hear.

He continued, "You might get pregnant and carry immediately until term, but you may not. You have to prepare yourself for a few failures before your ultimate success. What I suspect is that with each pregnancy, your double uterus will become stretched. Each time you'll carry the baby longer, until eventually you make it to term."

Simon moved closer and put his arm around me. We stood up, shook Dr. Mok's hand and thanked him for being a great doctor. He directed us to the receptionist to make our next appointment for six months later. We left his office with a dollop of hope that one day we would be proud parents, something we did not feel when we walked in.

The good news was that ten months after that appointment we received a positive pregnancy test. The bad news was that I had difficulties right from the beginning.

At eight weeks, I woke up in the middle of the night with blood-soaked underwear. One more time, Simon rushed me to the emergency room. There were two residents on duty and they both agreed that my pregnancy was in serious jeopardy. Coldly, they told me that I should prepare myself psychologically for a miscarriage. I did not want to accept their opinion and suggested that they phone

Another Day, Another Blessing

Dr. Mok. He told them not to do anything until he arrived. Dr. Mok entered my room and told the young residents that he did not agree with their prognosis. His intuition indicated that my progesterone was low and that was the main reason for my bleeding. From the shelf in the nurse's station, he pulled down a drug reference book. The hospital pharmacy did not stock the proper dosage of progesterone and he ordered the pharmacist to immediately locate it at another area hospital. Within an hour, the progesterone arrived and Dr. Mok injected it into my buttocks with this gigantic needle, which hurt when it pierced my skin. That was the first of two doses of progesterone spaced two weeks apart.

Progesterone is the hormone that prepares the uterus for the egg's implantation. I knew from hormone tests done as an adolescent (because I had excessive hair growth) that I already had a low progesterone level. Dr. Mok believed that if my spotting was due to a defective egg, it would abort itself spontaneously, but if it was due to a low progesterone level, then the injections would stop the bleeding and the viable egg would continue to grow inside of me. The bleeding stopped immediately. Our confidence in Dr. Mok escalated by the moment. He was our advocate and we sensed he would do anything to help me have a baby, even if it defied traditional western medical practice.

At 12 weeks, the cervical suture was inserted. This was done under local anesthesia. The next day I was discharged home, once again on Vasodilan to prevent any further premature contractions. Along with my daily multi-vitamin, I gulped those pills for the remainder of my pregnancy, afraid that missing one could cost me my baby—something I feared more than anything.

Because the suture was inserted after my cervix had begun dilating, I was summoned to bed rest for the remainder of my pregnancy. Our bedroom was located on the second floor of our two-story home in suburban Montreal. Each day at lunch, my dear friend Barbara and her five-year-old son, Karsten, mounted the 12 stairs with a tray of lunch, which Simon had left prepared in the refrigerator.

During those seemingly endless months, my writing hobby became both my work and my panacea. Simon built me a table and a ledge that swung over my bed, holding my typewriter. Each day, I recounted the events from the day before. My days were crammed with writing, reading, and knitting. The seemingly mundane events like receiving phone calls and letters became the highlights of my days.

Mild contractions or spotting continued to be part of my daily routine, as were regular visits to the emergency room, which ended up being at least once a month for the remaining six months of my pregnancy. Simon and I considered every day we had the baby as another blessing.

Our sixth wedding anniversary arrived on the 32-week mark. Simon was eager to celebrate and we asked Dr. Mok's permission to spend a day away. Because the baby was already viable, he consented. From a surgical supply store, Simon rented a wheelchair and popped it into his trunk and we drove to a luxurious resort one hour north of Montreal. When we arrived, Simon used all his weight training muscles to push me around the breath-taking rolling hills. What I remember most were the looks of pity from the other guests. The experience gave me a clear perspective of what it might have been like to be handicapped, even for just a day. By the end of our stay, I was pooped and Simon prepared the back seat of the car with blankets and pillows. At home, I crashed in bed from exhaustion.

At four o'clock in the morning, I was ripped from sleep by what felt like an ocean of fluids beneath me.

"Hon, I think my water just broke," I said, shaking Simon's shoulder.

His head ejected from the blue pillow much like those Jack-in-a-Box toys. He ran to my side of the bed, touching the sheets, and said, "Oh, my gosh. I can't believe it. We need to go to the hospital." Simon was so excited at the prospect of becoming a father that I think he actually forgot to lock the front door!

I reminded the attending resident in the emergency that my baby was in the breach position and that my obstetrician had already said I'd need a c-section. "I only want Dr. Mok to deliver it," I said emphatically.

"You're only a few centimeters dilated," he snapped. "We'll begin a pitocin drip to speed up your contractions and facilitate cervical dilatation."

By six o'clock in the morning, the doctors were fairly certain my baby would arrive soon.

My mind churned with thoughts as I lay staring at the white chipped ceiling. What about the risks of the newly-talked about A.I.D.S. virus? I wondered. It was

Another Day, Another Blessing

1983. The medical authorities were not yet sure about the effects of the virus, but had already advised hospital personnel to wear gloves when drawing blood. My instincts screamed out that my husband, as blood type O, the Universal Donor, should donate blood in case a blood transfusion was necessary during my cesarean section. He did, but thankfully I never needed a drop of it.

Eight o'clock the following morning marked the beginning of some intense contractions. The fetal monitor indicated that the umbilical cord was slowly tightening around the baby's neck. I was immediately rushed to the rather small operating room and given an epidural.

A curtain hung from a rod above the operating room table, landing on my chest, and cutting my body in two parts. It was impossible to see what was happening on my abdomen, the place where my baby would be brought into the world. Simon held my hand tight and all I could see were his gleaming eyes beneath his wire-framed glasses tucked between his blue bonnet and mask. Dr. Mok blurted out a rolling commentary of the events on the other side of the curtain. I shivered, fearing the worst.

"OK, the baby is about to be born," he said. Simon's mask stretched to accommodate his smiling face, and then the mask returned to its original position. The operating room became uncharacteristically silent. My husband's face moved to the other side of the curtain. We lost eye contact.

Did I give birth to a dead child? I wondered.

"Is everything OK?" I inquired. No one said anything. The seconds burned like hours.

The reason for the silence was that Rachel's color at birth was a dark shade of blue and the operating room staff was busy rushing her off for oxygen in the adjacent room. I felt so alone during those few moments lying by myself on the other side of that curtain, so cut off from what was happening with my body and my baby. Simon's head bobbed back and forth, from me to the baby until it disappeared completely on the other side of the curtain, as he helplessly watched the commotion surrounding our baby girl. Silence was interspersed with urgent requests for this and that. The few moments my daughter took to cry seemed like an eternity.

When Rachel Miriam was born on August 19th, 1983, she weighed a mere four and a half pounds. I had bought chickens larger than her. The nurses brought her to the premature nursery where she slept more than she was awake. In spite of my months of preparation, breastfeeding expended more of her energy than bottle feeding, so she pushed my breast away. I felt rejected and sad and this did not sit well with a new mother's ego!

Three days after Rachel's birthday, I spiked a fever because my cesarean incision had become infected. The nurses already knew to call Dr. Mok directly before even speaking to the residents. He immediately prescribed intravenous antibiotics. Because of the antibiotics, I was prohibited from visiting Rachel in the premature nursery. This news horrified me and I could not stop crying. To keep my milk flowing, I used this horrific milk pumping machine with a loud-sounding engine, which made me feel like a cow. After all that work, the nurses discarded my milk because the antibiotics would have been toxic to my baby.

During the day, Simon stayed near the hospital so that he could be present for the feedings. The premature nursery was just up the hall from the maternity ward. He shuttled himself back and forth from Rachel to me, always eager to help with us both, driven by the bliss of being the new father of a beautiful baby girl. Rachel and her dad developed a special bond during those days together.

After one week, I was discharged from the hospital, but unfortunately, Rachel had to remain there for an additional week, until she weighed at least five pounds, half a pound more than her birth weight. Our Aunt Lilly and Uncle Walter surrendered their city apartment so that during Rachel's second week we could be close to the hospital. I don't know what we would have done if we had to drive to our home a half hour north of the city during those critical days when Rachel was so fragile and her life so precarious. How could we ever get to the hospital quickly enough, if something had gone wrong?

On the morning of my discharge, Simon went to get the car, while the nurse rolled me to the hospital's main entrance in a wheelchair. Seated beside me at the door were other new mothers also waiting for their spouses. The only difference was that in their arms they held their babies. I looked down and touched my flat belly and knew that I had a baby; it was not a dream. A tear dropped on my cheek. Seeing those other women made me want to hold Rachel even more.

That night, when Simon and I lay down to sleep in the downtown apartment, we hugged and said how happy we were to have survived the difficult pregnancy. We rejoiced in the birth of our beautiful daughter, but we commiserated that there was an ominous emptiness echoing off the apartment walls, because our baby who had been growing inside of me for the previous nine months was somewhere else, being nurtured by someone other than us.

The days seemed like weeks as each morning we made our way the half a mile up the hill to the steps of the hospital. Not being able to hold Rachel whenever I wanted, combined with my hormonal changes during the postpartum period, made me prone to crying spells. I was very sensitive to anything anybody said. We were not religious, and I never prayed, but for the first time in my life I spoke to my beloved grandfather who had died three years earlier. I asked him to make sure that Rachel would be all right.

On the day Rachel was cleared for discharge, we made our last trip to the hospital. In her beige corduroy diaper bag, we put the little multi-colored sweater and hat that I had knit during my long months of bed rest. In her hospital crib, I bundled her up like I had done so many years before to my Tiny Tears doll. I wondered how it could be possible that this doll was real and ours—a little being who would be connected to us for the rest of our lives. We buckled her into her new baby seat in the rear of the car. I sat in the passenger seat, and for the entire drive home, my eyes were fixed towards the back of the car, admiring our new wonder and what a blessing she was.

That night, while tucking Rachel into the crib next to our bed, I was reminded again of my Tiny Tears doll and how many little girls around the world were tucking in their dolls and practicing for the real mom they will become one day. While watching Rachel sleep, I realized that every moment of bed rest, every moment of fear, every unexpected drop of blood, and the months of anxiety, everything was worth it—and that I would do it all over again, not once, not twice, but a million times, for just this moment of watching the most beautiful baby in the world as she slept.

19

Choice

Melissa Shook

There's a back-story to most events, including the birth of my daughter. Often it's not pretty. Mine wasn't. By the time I was 34 in 1973, I'd become capable of rattling off a short version of it to anyone I met. And most New Yorkers, trapped in traumas and patched together by therapy, also related a condensed version of their life stories so that once mutual confession was over, sympathy laced with humor could begin.

My spiel: My Mother Died when I was Twelve. I Lost almost all Memory of my Childhood before that, all sense of Her. My quiet Father Drank himself silly after marrying the nurse who brought my Mother home from the hospital to Die. I got Pregnant in college. Had an Abortion. Wouldn't have another when I got pregnant again. I wasn't married when I had my inter-racial daughter. She Is Wonderful. I had NO skills for making a living. It's been Hard.

It had taken years of therapy to learn to talk about these bare facts. It would take much longer to stop submerging my feelings, to set boundaries, and to start directing the course of my life.

I was born in 1939, 12 years after my mother and father were married. When I was eight, I accidentally overheard that she had been married before, and learned why my older brother had a different last name. When my mother died, her image was obliterated from my memory. I don't know what she looked like, how her arms felt when she held me, her scent, the sound of her voice, what her expectations for me were, if she loved me. I don't remember having lived within a family, of having been a child. However, I do remember the large house she'd chosen and carefully, if sparely, furnished. It was sold within a year of her death.

My father, a reserved mid-Westerner with a doctorate in math from the University of Chicago, was ill-equipped to bear the strain of keeping her four-year struggle with stomach cancer a secret, much less taking care of a 12-year-old. He quickly married Lou, the brassy nurse who had accompanied my mother on the plane home from the hospital and who took care of her for the last week she was alive.

Lou wore angora sweaters embroidered with beads. She wore falsies, tight skirts, high heels, lots of perfume, mascara, eye liner, lash thickener, foundation, powder, bright lipstick and crimson nail polish. This stranger, my new step-mother, carted me back and forth to visit her ex-second husband, an alderman in a Chicago ward, in whose bed she slept. Since she never told him that she'd married my father, Lou instructed me to call her by name in front of him and whisper "Mother" to her. I did not divulge her secrets to either man.

Over the six years she was married to my father, her visits to Chicago became longer while her stays at our suburban home on Long Island became shorter and less frequent. When she was away, my father drank tumblers of scotch and spent most nights sleeping in the bathtub. From my nearby bedroom, I could hear the water run in the middle of the night and assumed he'd turned on the hot tap, as if he were pulling up a blanket from the bottom of the bed because he'd gotten cold.

I took over the household tasks: washing and ironing my father's shirts, cleaning the house, opening cans of Chef Boyardee ravioli and heating frozen chicken pot pies. My frail paternal grandmother, a thin-lipped teetotaler, lived with us. She silently, but fiercely, disapproved of all the goings-on around her, most importantly, the demon drink. I bought my own clothes from money I earned as a popover girl at Lorraine Murphys' on Miracle Mile in the next town over. On the rare times my father and I talked, it was most often about writing—Edmund Wilson, Bertrand Russell, James Thurber, Francoise Sagan. We listened to Bob and Ray on the radio and very occasionally watched Sid Caesar and Imogene Coca on our small black and white TV.

Intuitively, I followed my father's example of being quietly understanding and unquestioning of all that transpired around us. He had taught me that conventional social norms are arbitrary and cloying, that religion is a leaky boat in which those wanting easy answers to the difficulties of life drifted, and that most everything is arbitrary, starting with the alphabet. I was raised as an agnostic because my father thought that the definition of atheism implied an argument about the existence of God, something he considered a "waste of time."

To compound what I'd experienced as a teen-ager, I chose the absolutely wrong college. Bard, a small liberal arts school located in an isolated area on the Hudson, was not the place for anyone as confused, repressed, silent and troubled as I was, though I had managed to appear like a fairly successful high-school student. I fancied that I'd chosen a radical school which would provide a rich climate for thoughtful, experimental study. That I was too emotionally damaged to profit from this intellectual stimulation was not apparent to me.

Too ill with ulcerative colitis to start college right after graduating from high-school, I spent the year in Manhattan where I began seeing the first of many psychiatrists. My father had rented a Greenwich Village studio apartment after selling our house, vowing never to cut another lawn. Only the bathroom, where he occasionally slept, had a door. As an escape from that situation, I took up with an Italian man, 12 years older, who saw me as a beautiful doll to be schooled in sophisticated culture starting with the New Wave of foreign films. He lived in a minuscule tenement apartment in Little Italy, shared with a fellow from Calabria.

By the end of that year, my father had divorced Lou and quickly married his third wife, a kindly, conventional woman with little understanding of his intellectual preoccupations or the complicated life he had provided for me. Now that he was in her capable hands, I went off to college, relieved.

When I arrived at Bard in 1958, I must have appeared to others as intelligent and attractive. My undoing was that all feelings about what I had experienced growing up were buried so deeply that it would be years before I understood anything of the toll upon me. I was numb to the core, but excellent at playing whatever role I thought was necessary to fit in. Only years later did I learn how common this "act as if" attitude is to those who have grown up in fractured homes or around alcoholics.

Many of my classmates came from equally troubled homes, but theirs were located in New York City. They had assumed a pretense of sophistication and were way ahead of the sexual revolution. Not for nothing was Bard nicknamed the "little red whore house on the hill."

By the time I quit school at the end of my sophomore year, having learned very little academically, I had slept with one icy guy who specialized in playing pool because his mother never let him forget that his older brother had tested at a genius level; a Hungarian freedom fighter who was dating the icy fellow's ex-girlfriend; and a drunk kid who, a few months after we had late-night-sex on the grass near the local bar, cracked up the flashy red sportscar his grandmother had just given him and died. Soon after that, I started dating Kemper, an ostensibly stable guy and an Army veteran. Unfortunately, I became pregnant. Very unfortunately. A few months before, a young woman had died in Queens after an illegal abortion. The newspaper headlines were ominous. Every abortionist had closed doors, shut off phones, including the legendary doctor in Connecticut to whose farm my friend had been driven in the dark of night the previous fall.

Kemper tried his best to find a solution, but there was none. Help, if it can be called that, arrived only after my father accidentally opened what he thought was a bill from the gynecologist and found out that I was pregnant. He called my psychiatrist who said that if two psychiatrists certified that I was too mentally unstable to have a child, an abortion could be performed in a New York hospital. My doctor was willing to write the letter, as was the severe European woman I consulted.

The hitch was that I was just over eight weeks pregnant, and since vaginal abortions were not permitted at that stage, it was necessary to have a hysterotomy, an operation not unlike a cesarean section. As I carried my small bag through the hospital lobby, I was positive that I'd die during the operation.

I didn't, and went back to Bard with a remarkable sense of optimism, believing that I had a future (though what it was I never pictured.) That feeling lasted about two weeks. At the end of the spring semester, I quit school to marry Kemper. Neither of us knew what we were doing, much less what we felt. I walked out on the marriage after six months, understanding nothing of the complex reasons that had lead me, us, to this crisis.

For four years, I drifted through unsatisfying affairs and tentative jobs, each paying less than the last. Then Darryl, a casual college acquaintance, phoned. He'd just been returned, broke, flown from Italy on an army carrier, courtesy of the American government. He'd been traveling there after graduation with a friend (ironically, the woman who later married my ex-husband) until her money ran out. I found him thrillingly attractive. His straight nose flared slightly at the nostrils, his cheek-bones were prominent, his chin sculpted, his skin a light tan with a spread of freckles across the cheeks, hair neatly trimmed into a close Afro. His easy smile showed a tiny gap between the upper front teeth. Darryl had the lean body of an athlete, a dancer perhaps. Those were the days when the term was Negro rather than black or Afro-American. He had been one of the rare non-white students on the Bard campus.

Flattered that he remembered me, I invited him to dinner at my St. Marks Place apartment, hardly imagining that once I'd opened the door, he wouldn't leave. After one night, we had begun living together. I never thought to protest. Only years later did I come to understand his profound passivity, to realize that he'd had nowhere else to go but his father's in the Bronx—a sorrier choice.

Darryl quickly turned the larger of my two almost bare rooms into a studio where he produced countless drawings on huge sheets of heavy paper—tangled charcoal lines, the center dark and hidden. Though his desire to paint seethed beneath the surface, he had no job and couldn't afford canvas and oils.

Perhaps because I had grown up with a father who parsed words, Darryl's reticence was intriguing. I imagined him a secret waiting to be revealed. I wanted to know what he knew, read what he read, think what he thought. When he wasn't drawing, he read books with glossy illustrations of work by Pevsner, Archipenko, Gabo and Duchamp, along with Klee's diary. I picked them up when he put them down and learned that devotion to the work was all that mattered; that artists were men and that becoming acknowledged was near-to-impossible, particularly for a black man. Who besides Romare Bearden had achieved recognition? I naively decided that his obvious talent—coupled with his highly valued light skin, handsome face, trim form and charming smile—would override any discrimination. The work that he somehow would magically produce would be recognized, exhibited and purchased.

Darryl never talked about the practical steps he needed to take to start painting, much less the problems that his race would have caused in having his work accepted to galleries. In fact, he only mentioned race twice during our seven years together. Once was to note that he habitually waited to enter our apartment lobby if a lone woman had preceded him, paused until she'd unlocked the inner door and started up the stairs.

Some months after he moved in, I became pregnant. Years later, I realized this was inevitable since I never checked my diaphragm. I didn't know how. The doctor's instruction to slide the rim behind or in front of or near some mysterious internal area was lost on me, though I undoubtedly nodded as if I understood him. I believed that women were responsible, the keepers of birth control. Condoms were something high-school boys saved in their wallets. I blamed myself.

I knew I wouldn't recover from another abortion. The pale, puckered scar from the slit into my uterus during the first one was a constant reminder of what had been taken from me. Though the mark had faded slightly in three years, a cyst of loss remained. My decision to keep the next child was made instinctively and beneath consciousness. It was not that I disapproved of abortion, but that my being could not tolerate another loss.

There was no joy in the pregnancy, but no sickness either. My stomach grew, the baby kicked, a doctor examined me regularly. Avoiding mirrors, I never noticed the forlorn expression that would have stared back. Darryl and I slept spooned together in the narrow bed, my face to the wall, and time passed while I waited to be delivered. I attended the childbirth class alone.

My father had raised me to question all conventions and never alluded to the fact that Darryl and I weren't married. This was apparently insignificant to him, though rare for the times. However, he chose a crowded restaurant at lunch time to say, "Have you considered what this baby might look like? Given the genetic mix, there is no predicting the color. Even if the father has light skin, it's entirely possible that the baby won't." Slave ancestors mixed with the genes of a white grandparent on Darryl's father's side and a Cherokee grandmother on his mother's allowed him to almost pass. My father's reasoning implied that I didn't know anything about Mendel's law. I did. It was irrelevant to me. My father wasn't overtly questioning my choice of having a child with a black man, but merely wondering whether I'd been fooled by Darryl's light skin into believing that it would predictably be of a similar color. At least that's what I assumed since the only prejudice he'd ever displayed, however mildly, was against religion.

I remember nothing of packing for the hospital, the first contractions, whether we took a taxi, only that the labor room was small and dark. I protested as the nurses shaved my pubic hair, put in the line for an IV. Some of the time Darryl sat on a chair while I lay there. I was surprised, since I thought he'd leave immediately and wait for a call.

The nurse gave me a pill she said would take away memory of pain. It did, leaving not even the dim recollection of early contractions. I stayed in this disassociated state until I found myself, child delivered, in a room with two other sleeping women. She was born on January 22, 1965, at 1:22 in the morning. I was 25.

My swaddled baby, tucked in a clear plastic cart, was wheeled in to visit me. Though relieved that she had ten toes, ten fingers, eyes which opened and shut, a strong cry, I did not allow myself to realize how lovely she was until Darryl visited early that afternoon and nodded his approval. Then I reveled in her pale skin, dark, straight hair and delicate features. Her brown eyes already appeared to focus. She looked ready for life. I have never lost the sense of how extraordinary she was, a vital being passed into my care.

"Shook, baby girl" was printed on the tiny white plastic wristband. We thought it would be a boy, Christopher Alexander, and had not picked a girl's name. I waited two days for him to decide on the name, Kristina Lisa, and to accompany me to the government office where he signed the papers and gave her his last name. I hoped this signaled his investment.

Choice

Because I had given up my pleasant apartment, believing the landlord would evict me for being unmarried and having a baby, we took her to a cavernous, low-ceilinged loft on the Bowery which Darryl had rented. In early mornings, a man's raspy voice called from the street below, "Don't forget to pray today, boys. Don't forget to pray." Looking down from the dirty windows, I watched a tall, shabbily dressed black man wave his Bible, exhorting men still sleeping in doorways.

Light from the front windows penetrated only a few feet into the dark, bare, cold space. Darryl constructed a small sleeping room in back with boards found on the street and insulated it with plastic sheeting. It was just large enough for the stove, the double bed he'd made from a discarded pull-out couch, a chair and the small table for Krissy's bed – my mother's laundry basket. A lamp burned day and night.

When he fired up the small wood-burning stove, the room briefly became so hot we took off all our sweaters, then cooled quickly. As I lay in bed and nursed the baby, I could hear the piercing sound of the power saw as Darryl cut firewood from trucking pallets he'd dragged back from trips around the neighborhood. I half waited for his screams, certain he would cut off a finger or slice his hand.

By the time Krissy was born, I'd already seen three therapists, but my reaction to any situation that might have provoked anger was delayed months, if not years. One leakage of what must have been buried rage against Darryl surfaced on the afternoon my half-brother came to visit. When I heard the doorbell and looked down the long, narrow flights of stairs as Darryl descended, I hoped to witness the blustering rage I'd occasionally seen my brother display, ungainly stamping and sputtering, his big face bright red: "What! What have you done to my sister, you good-for-nothing. How dare you....What are you going to do now?" I hoped he'd voice what I was unable to. Instead I heard his cordial greeting and watched he and Darryl chat amiably as they climbed up to meet the new baby.

Fears of death had long bobbed just beneath my surface. The only image I remembered of my mother was her skeletal form curled under a sheet on my parents' double bed shortly before her death. Often I crept toward Krissy's basket, later the crib, to reassure myself she was still breathing. When she was sick, I feared that the doctors would diagnose a serious illness. As she lay against me in the clinic waiting room, my racing heart must have transferred an animal sense of danger. By the time our turn came, three people had to hold the screaming baby down while she was examined.

In fact, Krissy's development was normal. She laughed and cooed, turned her head to follow a moving finger, reached for toys, arched her back and rolled over at the stages Dr. Spock deemed appropriate.

Darryl took care of her during the five or six hours I worked every weekday. When I discovered the ear plugs he'd been using while I was out, I worried whether he was feeding and changing her often enough, playing with her at all, but said nothing, having learned that questioning him was useless. Perhaps Krissy learned that crying when I wasn't there got her nowhere because she soon adjusted her schedule to mine, sleeping away the mornings, waking when I got home and remaining alert and curious until late evening when she finally accepted that the day was done.

Darryl refused to become a waiter again, a job he considered demeaning, and never searched for anything else. I was responsible for a baby girl and saddled with a man who didn't support himself, much less contribute to the household expenses. My employers, landscape architects, had accepted my unwed pregnancy, and they allowed me to work until just before the baby was born. I went back to pressing Lettreset and Zipatone patterns on presentation maps a week afterwards.

Consciously, I was captivated by the fantasy that Darryl and I were part of a collective change in America of the mid-sixties, not recognizing that our relationship was so detached and meager that we hardly functioned as a couple. Though I was virtually apolitical, never reading newspapers or voting, not owning a TV, friends had taken me to the Civil Rights March on Washington in 1963, where I'd carried a plastic bag with wet washcloths to breathe through if we were gassed. I'd been awakened by Martin Luther King's dream. In my mind, Krissy was riding the interracial wave, one of countless lovely mixed children of different shades, curly hair and beautiful eyes, lively and bright, harbingers of an equable association between blacks and whites. I gave not one moment's thought to what it would be like for her to bridge these two worlds, to be neither but both.

Choice

Understanding nothing of Darryl's background or the prejudice he'd experienced, I clung to the few stories he told about his childhood as emblematic. He told me of the brilliant satin costumes he wore singing in local talent events and on *Ted Mack's Amateur Hour,* easy success for the attractive, light-skinned boy. Until his voice changed. I visualized him as a young Harry Belafonte, so handsome and talented that he became accepted as a token by white audiences, in order to understand the expectations Darryl's mother had for her handsome older son. Her death from painful, disfiguring cancer of the jaw when he was 17 removed the support she'd provided as she willed him to become a successful black artist.

Krissy was little more than a year old the first time Darryl left us to catch a ride across country, to chase a dream in San Francisco. I sobbed as I listened to his footsteps descending the stairs from the sixth floor tenement apartment we'd moved into. This scene would be enacted many times when he came back and then left again. Sometimes, a letter from another woman on the west coast would arrive in my mail box. Occasionally, she'd call and I'd hand him the phone. I hadn't enough sense of self to be jealous.

Even though we were unhappy together and Darryl was emotionally distant and economically non-supportive, I longed for him as soon as he left. When he came back, things would be okay for a while, a few weeks, a couple of months, until I began to voice my needs. Once when I asked him to make dinner when I was late picking up Krissy from daycare after work, he said, "My people have taken care of your people for years. I won't do it." This bitter reference, only the second he'd ever made to race, silenced any more demands. The fact that Darryl acted out the same pattern that my father's second wife Lou had, of disappearing and returning, that I played my father's role of passive acceptance, continued until three years of sessions with my fourth therapist helped me sever my dependence on a man unable to love me or care for his daughter.

When Krissy was just weeks old, I started photographing her, recording her development, her father, our friends, the places we lived. At first, I knew nothing about exposing the film correctly, much less developing it and printing. I never imagined that a career teaching photography would slowly evolve from my obsession. At that time, I thought only of Darryl's work. Extra money pared from my small salary went for materials he needed: drawing paper, ink, charcoal. There was never enough to buy oils and canvas. I worried that he had so little.

It took four years to realize that I had started photographing my baby because I was unable to remember my mother. The few snapshots in the leather-bound family album provided my only image of her. It was not that I imagined that I would die and my daughter would forget her childhood in a tragic retelling of my own story, but I was still determined to create tangible proof of what she had experienced. When I began, I never imagined that I would photograph Krissy for 18 years until the morning she stood on the apartment steps for her last-day-of-high-school photograph and said, "That's it. You're finished with the series."

Those photographs chronicle the growth of my beautiful baby as she developed into a diminutive, sparkling, extroverted girl. Following my father's pattern of never telling her about my worries—the strain of providing for the two of us, my job difficulties—I also ignored talking about race. The moment she had the courage to bring the subject up is etched in my mind. I visualize the macadam street we were walking across when she said, "It would be so much easier if I looked half black instead of like I'm Irish. Why don't I?" She was already in high-school. Though she wouldn't have approved, I had been informing her teachers that she was bi-racial, that her first nine years had been spent in a dangerous New York neighborhood until she and I had moved to Massachusetts and that, for many years, her father played no role in her life. My hope was that this information would stop them from viewing her as the typical middle-class child, with two parents and a well-furnished home, like most of their students.

I would have died emotionally had I not given birth to my baby girl. Refusing to submit to another abortion was the first time I set a boundary, wasn't passively obedient to the needs of others. A big step. Through experiencing her alertness from the first moment I saw her, the way she later danced down our Lower East side block, her curiosity about languages spoken by strangers, the plays she invented, the stories she told, the costumes she constructed, I was given a sense of joy that helped lift me from the depression that had weighed upon me since my mother's death. Even though my childhood remains forgotten, my mother erased, my daughter taught me about life. Her birth saved me. Because of her, I had to grow up.

20

Millennium Baby Countdown

Martin Edwards

In the spring of 1999, my wife and I found ourselves pregnant. We were living in Brooklyn, New York, but since both our families were in California and this was our first child, we made the decision to move west. By December, we were mostly settled in a small house in the small town of San Luis Obispo. With most of our friends back East, and many family members scattered around the globe, I began to keep a diary of our birthing preparations on a website. This was before "blog" became an internet phenomenon, but I suppose that's exactly what it was. This was late 1999 and the media was simultaneously predicting the fall of civilization from Y2K bugs and the rise of an advertising juggernaut—the first Millennium Baby. Since the original due date of our child was January 1st—later moved to January 3rd—I called our diary the Millennium Baby Countdown.

Monday, December 27, 1999

Greetings from California, where the only way to distinguish seasons is by what's selling at the Gap. Christmas happened in leather. Happy holidays.

We are well-settled into our small house. Moving is an excellent opportunity to take account of one's belongings and shed the excess. The shedding will take the form of a yard sale, which will happen after the baby is born. I estimate a ten percent boost in revenue simply from having a cute baby hanging around.

Incidentally, the baby is healthy and exercising frequently in anticipation of its January debut. The baby's favorite workouts include boxing, rowing, and playing soccer—although we are puzzled as to where it got a soccer ball.

Tuesday, December 28, 1999

Last night we went to see *The Talented Mr. Ripley*. Jude Law is a very handsome guy and makes Matt Damon look a bit like chopped meat. Well, about half-way through the film, Lisa experienced her first contractions! This was bad timing on her part, as a crucial scene was playing out on the screen. Fortunately, Lisa used her relaxation training and was able to get through the film.

Pregnancy tip of the day: early, irregular contractions are known as Braxton Hicks contractions. While they do not signal labor, they are the first opportunity for a mother to experience what a contraction actually feels like.

Today we had our weekly appointment with Dr. Johnson, our obstetrician. He came highly recommended, with batteries included. Johnson's unique approach combines 27 years of professional experience with amateur night stand-up comedy. It's surprisingly effective for dealing with expectant parents, although I wouldn't recommend he play the Hollywood Bowl anytime soon.

We are happy to report that there's no protein in Lisa's pee, which is another way of saying that everything is progressing nicely. It's now less than a week till Lisa's due date, although we are constantly reminded that 85 percent of first mothers deliver a week or two late. It seems to me this pregnancy thing is a sloppy business.

We gave Dr. Johnson a copy of our birthing plan. It is a fairly detailed summary of how we want our birthing to go. When a teacher and a director have a baby, you can bet there's going to be a birthing plan.

Incidentally, *The Talented Mr. Ripley* is very good and we recommend it highly.

Wednesday, December 29, 1999

A lazy day, at Lisa's request. Made soup. Watched Alfred Hitchcock's *Marnie*. Found a couple more boxes to unpack.

Millennium Baby Countdown

But the highlight of the day was our final birthing class. For those of you who don't know, we have chosen HypnoBirthing as our method. The name is immediately misleading, because "hypnosis" carries a lot of baggage. I know I made several gold watch jokes before attending the first class. In reality, however, HypnoBirthing is about focus and deep relaxation. It is rooted in anatomy and working with your body to deliver your baby. And while the proof will be in the pudding, I am a believer. You have to be.

Thursday, December 30, 1999

We went to the beach today, and were treated to a spectacular sunset, replete with surfers and happy dogs chasing funny-looking birds with very thin legs. It was a special moment, until I realized we live on the coast and can pretty much do this any day of the week.

Still no baby, so Lisa and I decided to go on a date. With so much looming ahead—new year, new baby, possible apocalypse—we figured now was a good time for some quality one-on-one. We arrived at the restaurant, put in our names, and went to the bar. They don't smoke here, so what the bar lacked in smoky atmosphere, it made up for with maraschino cherries. As fate would have it, we sat down next to a pregnant couple. Due date? January 2nd. What a coincidence. We're January 3rd. We laugh. But wait, a third pregnant couple sits down next to the pregnant couple next to us. Due date? January 4th. Ha, ha, ha. At this point I'm looking around the room for the hidden camera and thinking this whole millennium baby thing has gotten way out of control.

The food was excellent, but more importantly, it had been a long time since the two of us had gone out alone, and we enjoyed that the most.

Friday, December 31, 1999

What if the baby isn't Y2K compatible? It'll pop out thinking the year is 1900 and grow up like the writer H.P. Lovecraft who, in his twenties, insisted that everyone call him "grandfather" because he was convinced he was born in the wrong era.

Spent the day partying like it was 1999. This involved watching a lot of CNN, just as predicted in the lyrics of the Prince song. That guy's a genius.

Negotiations with the baby continue, with the baby making no outward gestures of settlement. Is it mocking us? There have been no Braxton-Hicks contractions since we went to see *The Talented Mr. Ripley,* so this afternoon we went to see *Being John Malkovich.* An excellent film, but not worth recommending, since the ticket person informed us we were the last people on earth to see it. Alas, no contractions, although I did a fair amount of shifting—the seats were very narrow.

At 9 p.m., we watched Dick Clark's *Rockin' Millennium Special.* Although I wouldn't be caught dead in Times Square on New Year's, I became very melancholy. Peace to all our friends in New York, we miss you guys. Lisa and I welcomed 2000 with good food, drink and family, as planes crashed and financial markets collapsed around us. Better leave the clean-up for the morning. Happy New Year!

Saturday, January 1, 2000

Lisa made eggs for breakfast. As far as I can tell, there is no significance to this.

It is January 1st and the baby is not born. So much for those lucrative advertising contracts. And let us not forget that only ten percent of babies are born before their due date. So now all eyes turn to January 3rd. Have I mentioned that only fivve percent of babies are born on their due date?

Are Californians like lizards? The colder it gets, the slower they move? Because the temperature barely broke 60 degrees today and it was very quiet outside.

Was the highlight of today watching the *Whose Line Is It Anyway?* marathon on Comedy Central?

Sunday, January 2, 2000

A day of milestones. Lisa announced this morning that she is fairly certain the baby has dropped. This came as a surprise, as I was expecting a more dramatic event. "Dropping" refers to when the baby's head engages in the pelvis. (To whom the head is engaged we do not know, but we're sure they'll be happy.) In any case, the dropped baby has caused new pressure on her bladder and an occasional twinge sensation when the head presses against the pelvic floor. Alas, I do not get to experience any twinge sensations.

Lisa and I bought diapers today, a first for both of us. We both had big grins on our faces. We will mainly be using a diaper service, implementing disposable diapers for nights and daytime excursions. Of course, the purchase would have felt incomplete without a box of ass wipes. Is that what they're called? Well, that's what they do, so you get the point.

When we got home, we began packing the bag for the hospital. This is a big step. The birthing classes are complete, the baby room is coming together, and it's time to deal with the fact that the baby could show up on our doorstep any day now. I hope we get that three star rating from AAA in time.

Monday, January 3, 2000

No baby yet. Apparently, the memo informing the baby that today was the day did not arrive. No problem. We are, for the time being, infinitely patient.

Had our weekly appointment this afternoon with Dr. Johnson. The good doctor proclaimed he would put his money on a delivery sometime next week. He also took a keen interest in our website. If he checks out the site, I wonder how he will take being described as having "amateur night" humor?

We went for a walk around the neighborhood today. Spent much of the time noticing the peculiar plant life that inhabits these here parts, including the giant man-eating cacti.

Tuesday, January 4, 2000

First it was diapers, now pediatricians.

Today we interviewed our pediatrician, Dr. Maas, although "interview" is perhaps too strong a word. "Hung out with" is more accurate. Dr. Maas was surprised that Lisa and I are both the oldest siblings in our families, because older siblings tend to make nervous first parents who come into his office with long lists of silly questions. I agreed that first children often inherit their parents' anxieties, thus my model was to think what my parents would do and then do the opposite. Dr. Maas called me a genius. In any case, he's a cool dude with lots of experience and believes strongly in a mother's intuition.

Medical education tip of the day: Be a pediatrician. Kids are always being born, getting funny little coughs, getting things stuck up their noses—it's a growth industry.

Went for a long walk on the beach this afternoon then stopped at Splash Cafe for a bowl of clam chowder. Delicious.

Wednesday, January 5, 2000

This morning we looked over a checklist of things to do before the baby is born. Scored nine out of ten! We don't have our baby announcements yet, but that seems a little premature seeing how we don't have a baby. So, nine out of nine. Perfect score!

We went for a walk in the woods this afternoon. Walks have taken on great significance now that we've passed the due date, as they are considered good for inducing labor. Following a creek, we came upon a small bridge, ideal for playing Poohsticks, the game invented by Winnie the Pooh in the children's book, *The House At Pooh Corner*. Players line up on one side of the bridge, drop their sticks into the water below, and run to the other side to see whose stick appears first.

We tried a couple of games, but my sticks kept getting caught, so I soon found myself crawling under the bridge with a very big stick, clearing leaves and stones, and generally evening up the playing field. Thankfully, the water was not too cold, but even after this effort, my sticks continued to get stuck, and I was proclaimed the general loser.

Thursday, January 6, 2000

When one writes about one's life, especially when one's wife is about to give birth, one naturally runs the risk of a little banality. After all, to Lisa and I, simple acts like going to the movies or out for a walk take on absolutely thrilling proportions. And so, to all our readers out there who truly live dangerously, experimenting with Mongolese fusion cooking and attending Laurie Anderson concerts, I apologize, and give you... Lisa's shopping list:

Ipecac—Makes the baby throw up if it eats something bad, like an overdone steak.

Baby Nail Clippers—These things are really cute until you realize what you have to do with them.

Baby Tylenol—When your baby has the wrong kind of fever.

Nasal Aspirator—Babies don't know how to blow their noses. When Lisa first explained this device to me, I thought it was simply a straw you stick in their nose and suck. But it turns out there's a little squeezy ball at the end that does the sucking for you. Thank God.

Cotton balls—These fluffy, innocuous items are used for a horrible-sounding purpose... cleaning the umbilical stump.

Hydrogen Peroxide—Such a serious sounding substance. May I suggest a fun alternative—HydroPerx.

Small penlight—To check the baby's eyes for concussions, just like all the handsome doctors on *ER*.

Baby shampoo—Mild, mild, mild. So mild, I wonder if it actually cleans anything.

Friday, January 7, 2000

It's my birthday today. Perhaps not the birthday you're expecting, but come on, a guy's got to be born sometime. Hell of a day. Began with Lisa making me breakfast: cinnamon raisin French toast and bacon. Let me repeat. Cinnamon raisin French toast and bacon. Yes, that's right. Lisa rocks.

Then, around lunchtime, out of nowhere, my mother shows up. All the way from San Francisco. Totally unexpected. She had actually called in the morning to sing me "Happy Birthday." And then, four hours later, she and my step dad Glen show up at the front door singing "Happy Birthday" again. By the end of the day, she would find two more opportunities to sing "Happy Birthday."

Meanwhile, Lisa's been having contractions all day. They're wildly irregular, but who cares? It's something. Of course, with my mom around, it's hard to take it easy. First lunch, then coffee, then a walk on the beach. Finally, a respite before dinner, which Lisa spends laid out on the couch, watching the infinitely watchable *Win Ben Stein's Money*. Dinner was excellent, a procession of fine food and drink, followed by a walk to the (closed) video store. I like Captain Jack's Video, but no video store should close at 10 p.m. on a Friday.

Back home now, and Lisa's fallen asleep on the couch. I don't think it's going to happen tonight. But we could be close.

Saturday, January 8, 2000

Max, one of our cats, got in a fight last night. His back was so tender, he couldn't stand being touched. I wonder if the fight was with one of the chickens next door.

Lisa slept through the night, and today she experienced only a couple of small contractions. It was a let down after yesterday's performance, but we remain confident that the time is near. And she had a lot more time to rest today. My mum and Glen left after lunch, and Lisa was able to retire for the afternoon.

I wonder if our friends in New York are laughing at the fact that we have chickens living next door?

Sunday, January 9, 2000

This afternoon, we decided to see *The Cider House Rules*, the film adaption of John Irving's excellent, excellent novel. Lisa and I are both huge Irving fans, and I'm currently reading his memoir *My Movie Business*, a catalog of Irving's various experiences with having his novels turned into films, particularly *Cider House*. The movie is great (one of the finest book adaptations I've ever seen) and sure enough, half-way through, Lisa experienced some good contractions (something that I'd like to dub the Mr. Ripley Effect—see December 28 entry).

The contractions lasted throughout the evening, so around midnight, we started timing them. By the time we went to bed, at two a.m., they were relatively, consistently, approximately 15 minutes apart.

Stay tuned.

Millennium Baby Countdown

Monday, January 10, 2000 - 10 a.m.

The contractions continued through the night, and by this morning they were about nine minutes apart. Of course, I wasn't being a very good timer. Lisa would say "Now" when a contraction started. I'd look at my watch and then fall asleep in the next couple of minutes. I would wake up to a shove and Lisa's, "Now, I said, now." So we got up to have breakfast and more consistent timing.

Well, in the last couple of hours, the contractions have continued, but they're not exactly consistent. Nine minutes. 12 minutes. Six minutes. 10 minutes. What the hell is going on? So, good people, I ask you to remain vigilant. We have a scheduled OB appointment at 12:15, and I'm sure the doctor will have something to say. Like, "What are you doing here! You should be at the damn hospital!"

Monday, January 10, 2000 - 7 p.m.

Saw the doctor today at 12:30. He was very happy with Lisa's progress. The cervix is 100 percent effaced, which means it's as thin as it's going to get. Lisa's cervix has dilated noticeably over the last week. And, the baby has moved lower into the pelvis. Or else it has shrunk. And finally, the doctor guessed the baby would probably come in the next 24 hours.

The previous week's appointment had been so ho-hum, we were elated with all the things Dr. Johnson had to say about Lisa and the baby. We are now completely ready for the inevitable. The last thing to do was to shop for labor food—apple juice, chocolate pudding, apple sauce, chicken soup. Labor is exhausting, and incompatible with solid food, so you have to go liquid and mushy.

Yes, the hospital has a cafeteria, but a nurse warned us it wasn't so great. Nudge, nudge, wink, wink.

Oh, yes, the contractions. They're now lasting from 45 to 60 seconds, and anywhere from six to ten minutes apart. This is definitely progress.

More to come.

Wednesday, January 12, 2000

Okay, I've kept you waiting long enough. It's true, I'd rather sit around all day playing with my son than do anything else, and I thank everyone for their patience. But I'm now getting threatening e-mails and phone calls regarding the unfinished business of this diary. And so, without further delay, I give you the birth of Jeremy Robin Edwards.

When we last left off, it was around seven o'clock on Monday evening. Lisa's contractions were progressing, albeit erratically, and I had promised "more to come." Well, soon after posting this infamous entry, Lisa and I went over to dinner at her family's house. Amazingly, the topic of conversation was... Lisa's contractions. Of course, the whole family wanted to get in on the fun, and we soon had pen and paper out, playing "time the contractions" like a party game at an obstetrician's social mixer.

And then a funny thing happened. When I looked over the numbers, I realized the contractions had lost their erraticness. In fact, they had dropped to six minutes apart and were staying there. By this point, Lisa had excused herself from the table and was now relaxing in the lazy boy and breathing through the surges, which were now consistently 60 seconds long. It was becoming clear that the time was near. And so I resisted.

I resisted not because I was nervous, although the unknown tends to have that effect on people, but rather because I didn't want to jump the gun. Many expectant parents show up at the hospital much too early, and then sit around anxiously like stranded passengers at a snowed-in airport.

Hypnobirthing is all about relaxation. Lisa would be most relaxed at home, and I wanted her to have that advantage as long as possible. Of course, the contractions were now five minutes apart and Lisa's mom was reminding me that she'd had a few more kids than I had and it was time to go to the hospital. So I called the doctor to get his opinion. He thought it was a good idea to go in.

By the time we got off the phone, Lisa's contractions had dropped to three minutes apart. It wasn't a long phone call, it was just that the four minute contractions never showed up. Cheeky buggers. And so the reality of labor was upon us. I quickly went back to the house to get the car and suitcase and labor food.

The trip to the hospital was remarkably uneventful. San Luis Obispo is a small town. If we hit every red light, it would only take 5 minutes to get to there.

But knowing that there would be no dramatic in-car birth lent a certain serenity to the ride, while Lisa's family followed in the minivan.

When we entered the hospital, they tried to give Lisa a wheelchair, but she insisted on walking to her room. I remember saying, "If this is a false alarm, we're all going home." But I had nothing to worry about. The admitting nurse examined Lisa and announced that she was already four centimeters dilated. It was 10:30 p.m. and Lisa was in active labor.

We moved from the examining room to the labor room, which would also serve as the delivery room and recovery room. It had the feel of a hotel room— wallpaper, armoire, comfy chairs—with some medical equipment lying around, the sort of place I imagine Vegas lounge singers with emphysema spend their last days. The television had cable, and Juliet (Lisa's 16-year-old sister) was very impressed by the stereo system.

With the family camped out along one side of the room, Lisa continued to relax and focus through her contractions, while I attended her with a cold compress and massages. With Lisa focused on her body and I focused on Lisa, the next four and a half hours seemed to pass in half the time. Time distortion is a common component of Hypnobirthing, as is a shorter labor. In fact, our nurse was amazed at how fast Lisa was dilating. She twice had to reset her ETB (Estimated Time of Birth), from 6:30 a.m. to 4:30 a.m. to 2:30 a.m. As it was, full dilation happened before Dr. Johnson had time to get to the hospital, and for a moment, I think the nurse thought she would deliver the baby. By now, Tom had taken Lisa's two sisters home, leaving her mom curled up on a chair in the corner.

Just as Lisa was getting ready to make her first push, Dr. Johnson arrived. I suppose we all expected things to continue as quickly as before, but no one had taken into account that Lisa had never actually pushed a baby out of her before. Indeed, it took her a few tries to get the hang of it. Words of encouragement during the pushes, relaxed breathing and cold compresses between pushes, and one hour later, Jeremy's head popped out. I don't think words can describe that moment for me, so I won't bother. You'll just have to live with, "Jeremy's head popped out."

As soon as Jeremy was completely out, he was placed on Lisa's belly. Incredible. We just stayed there for a long time. At one point, after it had stopped pulsating, I was given the opportunity to cut the umbilical cord. Weird. Much thicker and tougher than I imagined - like a bicycle inner tube from outer space. But otherwise, we were left alone to spend quality time with our son. Three cheers to our doctor and hospital staff who followed our birthing plan to a tee!

Let me just take a moment to applaud the Hypnobirthing technique. Not only did it provide Lisa with the relaxation tools to work with her body, it educated us about the sociology and physiology of birthing, and the technicalities and complications involved. In fact, nothing happened that evening that I didn't understand or expect. If you're pregnant, or thinking about being pregnant, I would urge you to consider Hypnobirthing.

Well, that's it for the Millennium Baby Countdown Diary. Thanks for tuning in and giving us an opportunity to all feel a little bit closer.

Peace. Out.

21

The Zooming Birth of a Jett

Kiersten Forasté Shue

precipitate delivery / -sip -itit/, childbirth that occurs with such speed or in such a situation that the usual preparations cannot be made (Anderson 2004).

Mom's story
7:00 a.m.

As I mix the oil and cranberry juice I've substituted for the water to help slay the taste, I can't help marveling at the lava lamp like appearance of the creation. Unfortunately, petrol flavor cannot be disguised. I pretend it's exactly ten years and four nights ago at that college Halloween party where I was dressed up as road-kill (hell—I feel like road-kill right now but not as flat) throwing back shots of tequila. I manage to get the whole glass of morphing red castor oil down. The holistic women's remedies guidebook, recommended by my hippie friend, instructs the desperate pregnant woman to "Expect severe cramping and diarrhea to begin within one hour followed by the onset of regular contractions." O.K., so now I'll just lie next to my sleeping husband and wait for it all to gush through me.

One hour. Two hours. Four hours. Finally, my husband gets up and gets ready to head off to open his restaurant. I beg him to stay home since we'll be having our baby any minute now, but he reminds me I've been issuing that warning for a month. "No really, it's today... and soon," I plead. I can't tell him I've swallowed castor oil, he'll think I'm a freak. Who cares, it seems to have failed me anyway.

"I love you, and I love you, too (to the belly mound). Call if you need me. I'm right around the corner."

Ever since my OB visit three weeks ago, alarming me that I was already three centimeters dialated and 50 percent effaced, I've truly been expecting to just drop this baby out onto the floor every time I stand up.

Thud.

"What was that sound?"

"I don't know...Watch your foot, there's something on the floor. Oh, look! It's our baby!"

Instead, weeks dragged on until the discouragement was extreme, and having completed all imaginable nesting tasks and being a person accustomed to an obscene amount of excitement in life, the ennui became unbearable.

I watched 2000 episodes of *Birth Story* over the past two months in preparation for anything that may happen. I viewed shows with stoic women and thought, "I want to be like her! She's my hero!" And I viewed shows with demonically hysterical women, and I quickly pushed the record button on the VCR so I could show my husband later; that way, however insanely I labor, I'll appear a hero in comparison. During replay, I'd sneak peeks at his face to see how he handles seeing the sex, I mean *birth* canal as it spews clumpy blood. It's unclear, but he seemed to appreciate the scene as a miracle.

Every now and then I feel ashamed at my fear and self-pity as I think of pregnant African women. My brother is stationed for three years of Peace Corps service in a desert village in L'extreme Nord du Cameroun. He left just one month before I became pregnant. It's the first baby in our family, so I do my best to include him in the excitement by writing fairly detailed letters about the whole pregnancy. Alex writes me back letters about his work, cultural adjustments, and about two pregnancies in his village that parallel mine.

"One of my African friends, Moussa, has a wife who is expecting twins, and the village chief's third wife is expecting a baby, too...all three babies around the same time that you're due! These women sleep on hard bare earth surrounded by a few farm animals, if they are lucky enough to own any. At 5:30 a.m., they awake and begin to pound millet. By noon, the sun will be blazing at 120°F, and flies will sluggishly swarm everyone, so the women set off early on the 2K walk to the river to scrub clothing and fill their calabash jugs with water. The water is infested with flukes and amoebas, so everyone's always getting diarrhea and many children die. Moussa corrected me last week, 'It is impolite to ask a woman how many children she has because Allah has probably taken many and may take another at any time, but if you ask how many births she has survived, she will be proud. And don't be surprised if she answers 'twelve', or so!'"

I sent a printout of my 14-week ultrasound which clearly shows my shrimp-like fetus's skull, spine, and arms with five finger buds. The villagers laughed when my brother tried to explain in broken French and Fulfulde what the image is. Alex wrote back, "It is inconceivable to them that it could actually be a photo of your unborn baby. They think I'm a fool for believing your prank." Later, I sent a side-view photo of myself at eight months. "Now they are speechless. They wonder why you don't fall down with such a big belly on such a small woman. I saw a woman last week returning from the river balancing a full jug of water on her head, a baby in a pagne on her back, and her belly bulged a little. I'm getting to recognize the difference between a belly swollen by hunger and one carrying a baby, so I asked her how long she was pregnant and she said eight moons—same as you! I couldn't get over it! Her bump was almost nothing!"

Wow! So women (and girls) pray to Allah to let them live through childbirth and to allow the baby to live and maybe even grow up! Meanwhile, I'm swaying in my new glider rocker hoping that when the time comes, I won't forget to pack bottled water, that my epidural will work for me without intoxicating my newborn, and that my husband won't faint and knock over the doctor's instrument tray like my best friend's six-foot-four-inch tall husband did. I try to steer myself into keeping perspective, but it's like driving a car with terrible alignment, and soon I'm veering off track again into my own ditch of self-dejection.

So here it is, half way through the projected due day, and my big belly mound just sits obstinately on top of me. Castor oil failed me. Daily brisk walks failed me. A wave of panic washes over as I imagine myself a few years from now still pregnant and carrying a 50 pound five-year-old child. "COME OUT NOW you stubborn baby!" I admonish. He replies with a swift head butt to my bladder. He's displaced my kidneys, spleen, diaphragm, and everything else, so now I'm a mutated Picasso-like humanoid.

At one point during the day, I considered cheering up and taking Suki to the dog park in Charlottesville, a half hour away. After all, it's 65°F and sunny out. I imagine the torment of having to act chirpy to people I may meet there, and I opt for sitting around and muttering complaints to myself instead. Finally, I scarf down an obscene heap of macaroni and cheese.

6:00 p.m.

TWANG! GUSH! It feels like an elastic just snapped inside my pelvis. I jump out of my chair and stand there in awe, and slowly my thighs become wet. Then, OUCH! That birth instructor wasn't kidding when she said you'd know if it was a true contraction! Yikes and hooray all at once!

I call my husband and make a point to sound cool and calm, "Hi, Honey? I'll be needing you soon. I know dinner rush just started for you, so sorry about the timing. My water just broke, but take your time. They say the first baby takes hours of labor."

"Your water? What is the color, quantity, consistency, and odor?"

"Oh, Honey, I'm proud of you! You remember that from birth class? You're going to be...OUCH!"

Click.

"Honey?"

I get myself into the shower. I know I'll be a sweating spewing mess for the next great while, but I'd like to minimize the atrocity as much as possible for everyone who I want to be really nice to me. As soon as I step in, I become a writhing ball of pain on the tub floor. My husband is yelling up the stairs, "What the hell are you doing? Get in the car! Let's GO!"

The Zooming Birth of a Jett

6:30 p.m.

I throw on whatever with no shoes, dripping hair, and squirm to the car. As my husband drives, I call my doctor on the cell phone, but I can only eek my name and then some Satanic roaring sounds. Dr. Yoga* assures me he's on his way, too.

My husband attempts the it-could-be-worse approach by reminding me of the story about a Pakistani woman forced to labor on a high tree branch to escape drowning in a flood. I shut him up with a sound that mimics a rabid hyena tumbling into fan blades.

Halfway to the hospital, we're forced to stop at a busy intersection. I believe I've ignited into flames, so I roll down the window. The pain overtakes my whole being, and I begin thrashing my head from side to side—or perhaps it was spinning wildly on the axis of my neck, I can't quite remember, but in any case, I'm greatly entertaining the passengers in the cars alongside us. The rest of the trip is a blur, except for the part when the little blue Volkswagen bug in front of us decides to teach my husband a lesson for tailgating and slows way down. I scream like something possessed about how I'm birthing on our car's floorboards, and the driver of the bug swerves over to let us pass and to catch a glimpse of the laboring freak turning inside out.

7:00 p.m.

My husband arrives at the ER and expertly pulls into the ambulance-only semicircle. A burly security guard hurls me into a wheelchair and whisks me inside. The triage nurse dares to begin an admissions process. Between the grunts and shrieks burping from my mouth, I throw my wallet at her saying she can find my name in there and I'm pre-registered. She can't find me in the computer. "I work here, on the second floor, for crying out loud!"

Suddenly, like a Houdini team, my husband and a labor-and-delivery nurse arrive at once by my side. They ditch the admission and rush me to an elevator.

Now life is happening in flashes like a strobe light. I am in tune with the world around me for a few seconds, but then a tsunami of pain washes over and I'm delirious.

7:15 p.m.

In the room, the nurse leans forward to help me out of the wheelchair. Mmmmm. Her hair smells so clean. A voice says, "You're ten centimeters. Up onto the bed." I flop onto my back and wonder why they painted the walls such a dull beige color, then I realize that it's a beach mural.

"Too late for pain meds now. No, not even Tylenol, sorry."

More bits and pieces of reality frapped with excruciating pain.

My fragrant nurse says, "O.K., listen. With the next contraction, I want you to push."

I'm panicked, "But the doctor's not here yet!"

"It's O.K. We've done it before."

Then a man's voice. "Hello, Kiersten, or I should say 'Mom,' and hello, 'Dad'. It's nice to see you, again.

"What's with the pleasantries, Dr. Yoga? I'm tearing open over here!" Did I say that? ("No," my husband insists, later.) "I'm scared!"

"What are you scared of?"

"That my neurological pain pathways are going to short circuit and I'll die!" And I mean it. Bungee jumping in Taiwan wasn't nearly this scary; nor was meeting a 14-foot python in the wild Australian rainforest. Being held at gunpoint by rebel animists wearing goat horn necklaces and monkey tail belts in southern Senegal was the only contending experience. But this isn't an uncoupled emotional thrill; this, here, is real fear in response to real pain.

It's ironic how a calm and soothing voice can ring out above loud noise and chaos. And it's equally funny how a serene tone can feel like a grand slap. I hear Dr. Yoga's gentle voice say, "Kiersten, screaming won't help you push effectively."

I suddenly focus and realize this isn't a team sport. It's all up to me. "You're right. I can do this." I gather all my energy and ready myself to push it down into one fixed spot where Dr. Yoga is applying firm pressure with his latex finger to guide me. I explode with all my might into this feat. I'm powerful. I control destiny. I'm Moses parting the sea. I'm Superman rewinding time. I am a mother!

I am a mother! He praises me, "YES!—Wow! He has lots of thick black hair. If I had a comb I could style it!"

"Huh?"

But I feel another wave coming, so I gather and explode again.

7:31 p.m.

"Hello, Jett! Welcome, Little Guy!"

Pain and pressure dissipate. There's a lump of weight on my chest. I look down and see two dark eyes peering up at me. He's quiet, patient, tender.

Oh—it's still up to me. I should hold him. But I hear Dr. Yoga smattering about another push (to birth the placenta), cervical lacerations, and a second-degree perennial tear that needs to be stitched. My husband cuts the cord. Then a little needle pokes into my throbbing shredded vulva to deliver lidocaine, and I become numb. There's still so much commotion. I'm not quite ready to nurture my newborn son yet.

Jett passes his APGARs with flying colors and gets cleaned up. Although we named him at 22-weeks gestation, our baby has really lived up to his name in both English (born with the velocity of a jet plane) and Mandarin (recovering like a peaceful hero.)

Dr. Yoga continues his busy work of tugging and tying me. I want Jett's early moments to be filled with love and appreciation, and I'm just not there yet. So as he is held out to me again, I say, "Please let his Daddy hold him, first." I am lulled watching Daddy and baby, face to face, fully and peacefully taking each other in.

Jett's Story

We are driving home from our parent/child African Dance class. Jett is two years and three months old now. As we pass by Martha Jefferson Hospital, I excitedly pointed out the window, "Look, Jett! That's the hospital where you were born! You were a little baby inside Mommy's belly. Then I pushed you out, and you were a little baby, and Mommy and Daddy hugged you!"

Jett: "Yes, I was baby, and I kicked you."

Mom: "You kicked me?"

Jett: "Yes, I kicked and kicked you. Sorry."

Mom: "Where did you kick me?"

Jett: "In ya belly."

Mom: "Inside or outside?"

Jett: "Inside. Sorry."

I'm excited, but skeptical. He couldn't actually remember being in-utero, could he?

Mom: "Do you remember being inside Mommy's belly, Jett?"

Jett: "Yes."

Mom: "What did it sound like?"

Jett: "Heart. Boom Boom Boom."

Wow! This sets my heart racing. Could it be so? It's so hard to be sure of truths told by a 2¼-year-old. Last week I nearly burst into tears and raised hell when he told me something alarming about his sitter, "She's mean, and she bonked my head." Then he continued, "She flies around the house up, up, up at the ceiling with blue hair." I was thrilled about the possibility of Jett having true fetal memories, but in light of Jett's creative mind, I needed proof.

Mom: "Tell me more about in there."

...nothing...

O.K., Jett's verbal skills are very advanced for his age, but even so, expecting a descriptive monologue in response to an open-ended question is a bit too optimistic. The discussion had to be guided by "A" or "B" type interrogation.

Mom: "Was it dark or light?"

Jett: "Light."

Hmmm...

Mom: "Was it warm or cold?"

Jett: "Hot."

!!!

Mom: "Was it comfortable or tight?"

Jett: "Just nothing."

Mom: "Did you feel good in there?"

Jett: "Yes."

Mom: "Why did you come out?"

Jett: "Because I am was big boy."

I wonder if he remembers the experience of delivery with the fear and pain that I do. After all, his head coned into a squishy swollen cephalahematoma, a good inch tall for a good six months.

Mom: "Did it hurt coming out?"

Jett: "No."

Mom: "Was it scary coming out?"

Jett: "No."

Phew! Mom: "And who did you see when you came out?"

Jett: "Daddy."

I'd like to take credit for birthing my son; but in reality, I feel more like a force swooped down and pummeled me. My world was shaken to birth and raise this child. I guess from here on out, life will never slow down again. Jett was born with phenomenal speed and intensity, and now he attacks life with all he is and all he's got. I appreciate that. We do remember to putter every once in awhile—to recognize the discoveries, the frustrations, the hugs, the giggles as a succession of miraculous little moments—even as these moments in life try to zoom by.

Epilogue

The village chief's twins are two-years-old now. Alex tells me that, due to weakness and pain from malnutrition, they are not yet able to walk; and one of them whimpers continuously. Allah allowed the baby girl, heroically birthed by the other village Mama, to survive for three weeks.

Not my doctor's real name, but used in this story in honor of his peaceful aura, his curled guru-like mustache, and also in memory of the pretzel shape my body wound into during the pushing phase.

Sources

Anderson, Kenneth N and Anderson, Lois E. *Mosby's Pocket Dictionary of Medicine, Nursing, & Allied Health.* St. Louis, Mossoiri: Mosby, Inc, 2004.

22

Facing the Stars
to Silas on the occasion of your birth

Pam Rowen-Herzog

Silas, I don't really need to tell you this story: you lived it. It's buried deep, deep in your subconscious; it's an inseparable part of who you are. And even though it may seem foreign to you now, you will have relived this story many times, for this is a story of a journey from darkness to light. I hope by the time you read this journal, I will have told you of the mystery of the heavens embracing the earth more times than we can count.

May 10th, 2002, the day the books say you were due to enter this world, came and went. Your father and I were determined to let you decide when you were ready for such a brutal awakening, so we bargained with the midwives to let us go as long as possible before any intervention. But on Wednesday, the 15th of May, you began to stir and let me know that the day was coming soon. I woke up Thursday morning with an overwhelming desire to stay cuddled up in our dark orange bedroom, light some candles and turn the heat up on high. So I didn't go to work. I hibernated, but nothing happened. The same thing happened Friday morning when I woke up, so I indulged again and prepared my den.

Daddy came home from work around 1:00 that day to take me to an appointment at The Birth Center. Now that you were one week overdue, the midwife insisted we begin some natural induction methods to send you a message. But by the time dad arrived home, you were the one sending the message—

166

contractions were coming every five minutes. So we anxiously drove to see the midwife and she indeed confirmed that we were in active labor. Overcome with joy, your dad and I decided to go shopping for a rocking chair for the back patio. I was dreaming of spending lazy summer evenings on the back patio nursing and rocking you to sleep. So we drove from store to store for the next few hours, every five to ten minutes stopping so I could lean against your father. He'd whisper encouraging words in my ear as I took deep breaths and rode out the pain.

That night the contractions slowed down a bit and became less intense. Neither of us slept much as we anxiously anticipated your arrival. However, Saturday also came and went with little progress and only periods of intense pain. We took walks and I bounced on the birthing ball while listening to African drummers, but mostly we stayed cuddled up in the third floor bedroom with only candles lit. Your dad meticulously recorded the length of each contraction, the length of time in between them, and their intensity. We had decided that we wanted to be home for most of the labor so we were waiting until the contractions were consistently 2 minutes apart before we would go to The Birth Center. But you still were not ready to come.

Then around midnight on Saturday, you became much more serious about your journey to this world. Daddy was exhausted and needed sleep. I was also exhausted and slept in between the contractions, which were now coming every seven minutes. They were so intense and combined with my exhaustion, they seemed unbearable. I passed the night sometimes laying in bed and other times sitting on the birthing ball listening to whales on a borrowed CD from Aunt Lisa. The whales groaning were so eerie that I figured they must be conveying compassion for me. They cried with me as I cried with pain and as I imagined you struggling with your entire little infant might to fight your way through the narrow canal.

During each contraction, I would say to myself, "I can't take this anymore; I must wake up Bob." But I was so spent that by the time the contraction started to subside, I would lay my head down on the bottom of the bed and fall asleep only to be rudely awakened six minutes later. Your father woke up every hour when I went down to go to the bathroom and asked how I was doing. I only had enough energy to say that it really really hurt and drift off to sleep again.

This dark Saturday night was the beginning of the meeting of heaven and earth, like nothing I had ever experienced before. With each contraction, I felt Mother Earth suck me down into her black hole where I joined the 300,000 other women and millions of animals around the world giving birth that day. My groans were part of a harmonious chorus. They were otherworldly, and joined the song of the Life Force that is humming continuously throughout all time. I wanted to surrender completely to this black hole but I resisted. It was too unknown and the pain too great. So with all of the survival instinct I could muster, I fought it.

By 7:00 a.m., I was at my end. Daddy woke up and we decided to call the midwife even though the contractions had only progressed to five minutes apart. She said if it would make me feel better, I could come in and she would check the status of my cervix. So at 10:00 a.m., we packed our bags in the car, picked up Grammy, and headed in. With each contraction, I cringed and grasped daddy's hand. When we arrived, Denise was the midwife on duty. She asked us not to unpack the car until she measured my progression; I could not bear the thought of having to go back home again. Fortunately, the exam showed that I was five centimeters dilated, "a keeper" as she labeled me. Grammy unpacked the bags and we moved into the front suite with flowery wallpaper and a big double bed.

With the good progress report came a surge of energy and excitement. I couldn't sit still and paced the small birthing quarters—around the living room in circle after circle, through the kitchen, into the bedroom and back to the living room to circle around again. The exam had also shown that you were face up, posterior, or "sunny side up" as they say. I remembered in birthing class that this was something to be avoided if at all possible because it causes dreadful back pain and slows down labor and delivery. However, Denise was very calm about the discovery, certain that we could turn you around, so I did not worry. During each contraction, daddy stood behind me, placed his hands on my hips and helped me to rotate them as I bent my knees and leaned against anything available.

After a couple of hours, Grammy ran to the store to get lunch and I soaked in the hot tub. She had picked the first lavender clematis of the spring from her back patio for me, so I clung to this sign of life during my bath. I tried to imagine myself opening up like a flower with each contraction. I pictured you scared yet determined to make this journey, showing more courage than most grown-ups I know. I could feel that we were a team, you and I, pressing on, laboring to meet each other at last. My water soon broke in the tub and it was time for another exam. It revealed that you had turned half way and I was now nine centimeters dilated. So I paced the suite again. Contractions hurt, but walking, lunging, and daddy's encouraging assistance helped to keep my spirits high.

Then my contractions began to slow down. Another exam around 2:00 p.m. showed that you had turned back, so you were once again facing up. This meant you were having an incredibly hard time squeezing through. I was dilated to 9 ½ centimeters, so we concluded that this was the way you had decided to come into this world, with your face toward heaven, facing the stars. Daddy and I were extremely committed to a natural birth, believing that even though this was the harder road, it was a great gift we could give to you. We trusted your body and my body, that, barring any extreme emergency, God had created us to work together in harmony to bring about life, your life. So we buckled down for the ride.

Denise was concerned about my uterus stopping altogether since it was completely exhausted from the already 49 hours of labor. So she enlisted daddy to do nipple stimulation, producing oxytocin which causes contractions. It worked and once again this Life Force began calling to me. I tried sitting on the birthing stool with daddy sitting on a chair behind me, but because of your position, my legs kept falling asleep. So I had to lie down on the bed propped up against your dad. Marie, the nurse, entered to assist. Soon the black hole became more real to me than the flurry of activity in the room. With each contraction, I descended while desperately trying to stay connected to this world.

At one point, I remember daddy breaking down and crying on my shoulder. I felt as if he had gone to the edge of the abyss with me, looked straight into it, and watched me fall. All I could scream was, "It hurts so much," as I feared I was being consumed. But his tears showed that he had heard me, which in turn gave me more courage. By this time my connections to this world were brief but vivid

—Grammy putting a cold wash cloth on my forehead or holding a bucket while I threw up.

At 3:00, it was time to push you out. During my pregnancy, I had romanticized this transitional moment, believing the climax was right around the corner. But here it was and I had no urge to push. In fact, I didn't even know how to push. Each time a contraction came, everyone in the room would yell, "PUSH!" and I would tense up my whole body. Denise kept saying, "No, push into the pain." After awhile, I remember her sternly telling me that I had one more push and if I didn't make any progress, she was going to give me pitocin, a drug to help my uterus contract. At these words, I re-entered this world enough to process her direction of pushing into the pain. I realized my resistance. When I relaxed and pushed, the pain was so unbelievable in my lower back that I would tighten up my whole body to avoid it. But that was exactly what was keeping the birth canal closed. My fear, my resistance, was blocking the way to life. I needed to surrender everything to the Life Force, entering even further into Mother Earth's black hole, not knowing whether or not the pain would consume me.

For the first day and a half of labor, I had been able to ride the waves of contractions without drowning. But during the pushing phase, the waves were too large to control. It felt like body surfing in the ocean. If you catch a wave just right, you can ride smoothly on top. But if you don't, you only have two choices. You can either furiously flap around trying to swim and stay afloat, or you can take a deep breath, relax and let the wave wash you wherever it wishes. Only the latter works, because if you don't surrender to this force that is larger and stronger than you are, then you end up gasping for air, flailing around, and possibly getting injured. But if you surrender to the currents of the wave, you can curl up, trusting that it will soon be over and that you will come to the surface for air once again.

So I stopped arching my back, relaxed, and let the next contraction—a tidal wave—wash over me. I pushed into the pain, into the unknown, with my whole being. And sure enough, not long after, out emerged a tuft of black hair! Denise called daddy and Grammy over to see, and I will never forget the indescribable joy and exhilaration on their faces at their first glimpse of you! It brought me billowing back to this world. I had surrendered to the darkness and felt life emerge. You were on your way.

The tone and the energy of everyone yelling "push" changed. It was now charged with such excitement and anticipation that it joined the chorus of all living beings being born at that moment. This world had merged with the spiritual world. So with the song and energy of your daddy and Grammy, I pushed, and you struggled and squirmed until you—Silas Emmanuel Rowen-Herzog—entered this world at 4:50 p.m., May 19th, 2002.

You appeared with your head held high and proud, your first glimpse of this world toward the heavens as you had determined, and covered with long dark hair. Your broad shoulders got stuck, but after Nurse Marie gave one sharp push on my belly, you popped out. Your father and I sobbed.

You took right to my breast. You knew me, my heartbeat and the rhythm of my breathing. We were one again, at peace, slowly waking up to this new world together, both emerging from darkness into light.

Your father and I laid in bed with you in speechless wonder. Grampa arrived and Grammy made a celebration dinner; I was as hungry as you were. After dinner Grammy brought in a chocolate cake with the spring's first ripe strawberries on it, yet another sign of life. It had a big zero candle on top and we all sang "Happy Birthday" to you, continuing this Song of Life. I bathed; you weighed in at eight pounds and 11 ½ ounces; and daddy rocked you to sleep bare-chested. By midnight, we were packed up and headed home, a new family. We were bursting with love for you, for what you would become, and for the mother and father you would mold us into.

I felt like I was covered with a sacred glow. In the Hebrew Scriptures, it says that a mother is unclean for weeks after giving birth. Uncle Chuck says there is a tradition that speculates this may be because labor and birth bring a woman so close to God—to this burning, consuming Life Force—that she is then dangerous for others to be around. Maybe it is not so unlike Moses when he came down from Mt. Sinai and was glowing after his glimpse of God.

"In the beginning God created the heavens and the earth. The earth was formless and empty, darkness was over the surface of the deep, and the Spirit of

God was hovering over the waters. And God said, 'Let there be light,' and there was light. God saw the light was good, and God separated the light from the darkness."

Silas, you were born out of this darkness, this depth. You entered this world through the paradox of God's creative love—life from death, light from darkness, the collision of this world with the unknown spiritual world. May your life journey always reflect this divine mystery as you continue to face the stars.

I love you. —Mommy

23

Letting Go

Sarah Briggs

"How *much* water?" That's all our friend Dawn heard when she suspected that Norm would be heading down to the emergency room that night. She still makes us laugh when she tells her side of the story and mimics her husband's query. I had been lying in bed at about 11 at night, just drifting off to sleep, when I felt a sharp, low kick and a gush of water flowing out between my legs. I was stunned at first, realizing on a deep, visceral level exactly what had happened, but reassuring myself intellectually that it couldn't be my water breaking as it was a month before my due date. I told my husband in a nervous and dumbstruck voice that some water had spurted out, and we both considered going back to sleep, to allow the labor to progress at its own pace; but we called Norm, our good friend and pediatrician, to get another opinion. He was reassuring and suggested that we call the hospital, since my midwife was out of town for the weekend. The nurse on duty in the newborn wing advised me to come in to check the baby's condition, saying that she would call my doctor and that we'd figure out the best way to proceed from there. I felt a wave of dizziness and fear, which surprised me. I had naively figured that I'd be confident and yet flexible enough, mentally and physically, to deal with whatever happened. How many times had I meditated on acceptance and the chance nature of life, so full of change? Yet here I was, feeling that all-out-of-control rush I'd hoped to avoid. The lessons of motherhood had begun! It was one thing to tell myself intellectually how I'd respond, and quite another to experience the panic that arose because my body was entirely and solely in charge.

Having planned for a natural birth, I hadn't discussed other options in great detail with my obstetrician. I had been in for one of my normal prenatal check-ups just two days earlier, and had found out for certain that the baby was still breech. I had suspected that at the last check-up; but it was a different doctor that day who thought the baby had turned head down, and, unfortunately, I lent his opinion more credence than my own intuition. Once I knew that the fetus was still feet-down, I began to lay at an incline with my feet up for 15 minutes twice a day, in a gentle effort to help the baby turn around. I had felt heightened activity in the womb, but nothing had changed, and we didn't have time to try any other manual turns. This was exactly when I needed advice from Marta, my midwife. She worked in tandem with my doctor, and was the one I had best connected with emotionally and spiritually, whose centered voice and calmness I knew I could rely on to help me get through the worst moments. I enjoyed the prenatal yoga class she taught, trusted her knowledge, and appreciated her openness about her own birth experience. She knew how much I wanted to do the bulk of the labor at home and only go into the hospital when I really needed to towards the end. So as we drove the five minutes to the hospital, I was afraid it wouldn't be the type of birth I'd hoped for and knew that I would sorely miss Marta's help.

If I had been younger than my 42 years or had had another child before, I would have insisted on a home birth. That seemed the best way from my perspective, after reading books and talking to other friends who had given birth at home, in birthing centers, or hospitals. I had taken several lessons with a Bradley Birth Method teacher and knew I'd be most comfortable psychologically at home, thus, I hoped, more relaxed and able to grapple with the intense pain. I imagined relying on my hours of meditation, pushing through discomfort and pain both on the mat and in sports, as well as some of the breathing ideas and postures I'd practiced, music I love, and the encouragement from Scott, my husband, and Marta. I was looking forward to the unknown, as a test of endurance and acceptance. But Scott was terribly uncomfortable with the idea of going through it at home, and there was no birthing center in the small town where we live, on an island in southeastern Alaska.

Our other major concern was that I have a history of manic episodes. I had never gone through a serious depression, but was labeled bi-polar after my first psychotic break in 1988. I had been off medication for nearly ten years and hadn't had any problems until the spring of 2000 when I participated in a week-long Zen meditation retreat, or sesshin. I knew that it was a bit risky, given my sensitive brain chemistry, to attend a retreat where I would be getting up at 4:30 each day, eating less, and trying to glimpse a state of samadhi, defined by Philip Kapleau as "not merely equilibrium, tranquility, and one-pointedness, but a state of intense yet effortless concentration, of complete absorption of the mind in itself, of heightened and expanded awareness." Lack of sleep is one of the factors that can easily contribute to my hypo-manic mood, which can then escalate into a full-blown psychosis if I ignore my rising level of excitement and energy. I had trusted that the meditation and breathing would ground me, but was unprepared for the amazingly sharp insights I began to experience. Flowers suddenly seemed to have an extra dimension, the vibrancy of colors, smell and texture jumping out at me in indescribable beauty. The answer to one of the koans (illogical puzzles) we studied popped into my head, even though I wasn't officially working on it yet. I felt an immediate and exuberant connection to the world, which was exactly what I had wanted. I had no inclination to staunch that powerful flow of sensations. That's the dangerous allure of mania—just when I feel most alive is when I begin to slip away from "reality" as most people see it. Would the intense pain and sleep deprivation of a long labor, and the overwhelming joy and intensity of birth, push me over that edge again? After several months of deliberation and weighing the options, I agreed to give birth in the relatively low-intervention hospital here in town.

I soon found myself in the position I had promised I would never be in—lying down flat in a hospital bed, attached to a monitor. Since so much water had escaped very quickly, my doctor insisted on that procedure to follow the baby's heart rate and to check the baby's position. I hated being strapped in like that, hearing the incessant beeps and whirrs of the machine, inundated by an antiseptic, metallic smell. But I was mesmerized by my belly—it looked as if the baby were shrink-wrapped inside of me, my skin smooth and taut, with the outline of the baby's body protruding in an oddly clear way. The nurse asked if I felt the contractions, and I was honestly able to smile up at her and say that I barely felt anything yet. My doctor did an ultrasound and determined that the baby was breech, with one leg up and one leg down. She discussed our options with us and, although she was patient and clear, I sensed immediately that the choice was not really mine at that point. Since it was my first birth, she felt that a breech delivery would be too risky, particularly given the baby's current position. I didn't express my frustration, but I was thinking that she simply hadn't had the opportunity to do enough breech deliveries, and that if hospitals didn't intervene with so many cesarean sections, breech births would be considered more routine and less dangerous.

Lying there as the labor pains became more intense, certainly noticeable by now, I had trouble focusing on what she was saying. I was mildly alarmed at how quickly the cramping had become deeper, and was unsure how I would handle another several hours of increasingly sharp pain (not to mention the "rocket blast" of pushing out a baby, as one of my friends had described it…). The doctor was ready for us to agree to a cesarean, and I saw Scott slowly nodding his head. Thinking back on that moment now, I honestly can't say if I felt more a sense of relief or disappointment—my feelings were all jumbled together and my brain was foggy and confused. It did seem the best solution, as I wasn't up to arguing with a fine doctor whom I trusted and who knew how much I had hoped to have a natural birth. If she didn't think it was a good idea to try, I had to go along on faith that her judgment was more sound and based on far wider experience than my own. It was clearly the safest choice for the baby, so I made my decision quickly once I accepted the situation and let go of my desire for a birth that wasn't ever going to happen in the way I had hoped. I did have implicit confidence in my doctor's ability as a surgeon, so I was pleased to have her take charge and was ready to get on with the operation.

Thus, barely three hours after my water broke, a nurse had wheeled me down to the operating room and I was receiving anesthesia through my spine. I had been through an epidural two years previously after I broke my leg badly, skiing, (skiing badly), so I wasn't quite as nervous about it as I would have been otherwise.

Letting Go

Forcing myself to try to sit absolutely still as the needle stung and entered required some concentration, but it was over quickly. It reminded me of having an eye exam when you know the opthamologist is poking your eye with a needle to check pressure for glaucoma, and you're hoping like hell you don't shake or move and rip your eyeball! I didn't let myself imagine what would happen if he hit the wrong part of my spine; I told myself that he had done it over and over and this was just one more job for him. I was also prepared for the active, loud noise level and jarringly bright lights in an operating room, so I was less disturbed by that then I had been the first time. I'm squeamish at the sight of blood, so decided not to watch the proceedings through a mirror and only imagined what was going on behind the screen they had erected on my belly.

As the doctor cut me open, she explained that they do it below the bikini line so that the scar isn't as offensive—which was the last thing on my mind at that moment. Scott also opted not to watch, so he was beside my head, stroking my hair and holding my hand as it became uncomfortable. I was staring up at the lights overhead and commented to him that the light coverings were almost blue-hued, and that was better than buzzing, vibrating fluorescent lights. I felt strong tugs and very unsettling pulling, and I was trying not to imagine my intestines being pulled out and organs pushed aside as the doctor tried to move up into the uterus from so far below. She remarked that my abdominal muscles were extremely tight as she continued to yank what felt like muscles and tough, fibrous tendon. She wrestled around inside of me for what seemed a very long time, and I wanted to shout, "Is everything okay down there?" Instead I gritted my teeth, squeezed Scott's hand harder, and focused on how much I like my tight abs.

Just as I was hoping it would be over soon, she said she was "there." I felt a huge emptying and release, and then the room filled with loud crying and Scott moved down to take the baby, announcing that we had a boy! The emotion in his voice contained everything that I love about him—gentle tone, yet full of depth, somehow both calm and joyous. Before the birth, I had imagined that the crying would be upsetting. Yet as it happened, I began to cry and laugh with joy-filled relief to hear powerful, healthy lungs and a gusty infant wail that any parent can recall—high and thin, louder than seems possible from such a tiny body.

I had hoped to breastfeed immediately, but they were not equipped with enough space to allow that on the operating table, and they needed to put everything back inside of me and close up the incision. So I held our son for a brief time on my chest, watching his face and perfect little body in amazement, his reddish gray, slippery-wet skin not ugly to me at all as it had seemed in photos and films I'd watched. As my husband and the pediatrician took our newborn son upstairs to clean him and weigh him, I lay on the operating table, feeling rather abandoned as the doctor joked with the nurse and anesthesiologist about golfing. I was in a completely different space, still reeling from the speed of the delivery. My mind was in post-miracle haze, with thoughts of not having an infant car seat or a changing table bouncing around with images of my parents' faces of delight at the news and knowing now which of the two chosen names we would be using: he would be Stone Briggs Cornelius, and Elaine would remain just my mother's and my middle name.

As soon as I was ready, they rolled me upstairs to my own room where I spent the next two-and-a-half days bonding with our new baby. The nurses were so helpful as I learned to breastfeed, and I quickly lost any embarrassment I felt in having one of them squeeze my nipple and put it deeper into Stone's grasping mouth. He had a hard time latching on properly at first, and when we finally got it right, I had another surprise—*Oh, THAT'S how it's supposed to feel!* The sucking was much more intense than I had been imagining. It was a rush of pain and then pleasure as I got used to the novel power of his vigorous little mouth and tongue.

I liked the feel in the newborn wing; many of the nurses were ex-hippies with relaxed and genuine manners. I struggled with a horribly itchy rash from the morphine, and the nurse on call eased my discomfort by massaging lotions onto my back and opening the window for me despite the cold outside temperature. The night nurse carried Stone around in a sling so that he was never left lying in an incubator while I tried to sleep. After an almost sleepless night and the round-the-clock nursing, I was a bit concerned about the possibility of becoming manic. I was upset when I realized that the rhythmic contracting and releasing of the morphine drip was too loud and insistent for me to ignore, and I began to hear words along with the noise it made. That was often a first sign of growing psychosis for me.

Letting Go

When my doctor visited me later that day, I asked if she could please turn off the drip pump and put me on any other type of pain medication. I knew I could deal with pain better than nausea after my broken leg. I was frustrated with her response, looking at me matter-of-factly and saying, "We usually leave it on for 24 hours," as if she hadn't just heard me voice my specific worry and request. It was only after Scott, who is a psychologist, spoke to her about his concerns that she ordered the nurse to disconnect the drip. What if he hadn't been there as my advocate? Why didn't my opinion matter or carry as much weight in her eyes? Fortunately, as soon as the pump was disconnected and quiet, I was able to sleep better and returned to the more normal state of new-mother exhaustion, with no overtones of mania. My elation was grounded in daily discoveries with Stone and Scott, and it helped carry me through the irritation of, to my mind, invasive hospital routines.

As I told friends about the birth in the days to come, I realized how disappointed I was at the many missed opportunities. I had wanted to be brave and pass the womanhood test with courage and honor. When other mothers told me, I suppose to console me, that I was lucky to have missed all of that agony, I felt guilty at having had such a speedy, relatively painless delivery. I only accepted it when I heard similar words from a friend who regularly runs marathons and is an amazing athlete. She can endure enormous pain and has stamina and heart to get her to the finish line, qualities I admire and try to emulate. It was only then that I began to accept the birth exactly as it had happened, and gradually to be grateful for it as well.

Now, 15 months later, thrilled at having a healthy, running, talking, laughing little boy around the house, I know that I can continue to reinvent the story in my memory. Memory is part fiction as well as factual truth, because it's not just my story, but my husband's and son's as well. I don't want to negate or minimize my own subjective experience, but I can expand it by melding other memories into that one strand of truth. While I was lying there feeling cut off and dazed, Scott was carrying Stone, in that tentative yet firm new-parent hold, and beginning his own bonding as a father. He laughs at how our beloved, warm, and sometimes absent-minded pediatrician friend led them all up the main elevator instead of a side one, so that they emerged on the long-term care hallway instead of the obstetrics ward. The nurse at the desk gave them a reproachful glance even before the baby began another Banshee-like cry, no doubt waking up most of the patients nearby. Scott recounts with a grin that when they finally arrived and were cleaning him off, Stone's left leg was splayed up by his ear, having been stretched up in that position for many months, proudly showing off his big, distended balls to the world! I realize that I can stop mulling over and over the petty losses I felt after the birth. I'll become more who I want to be if I remember, rather, my amazement and surprise and elation, if I close my eyes and hear again that newborn cry, recalling and reliving the bubbling wonder in my heart.

Source

Roshi Philip Kapleau. *The Three Pillars of Zen.* New York: Anchor Books/ Doubleday. p. 376.

24

Arrows

Sabrina Porterfield

"You are the bows from which your children as living arrows are sent forth."
Kahlil Gibran

Mama. Woman. Scarred warrior.

On my belly, proof of my nine month long crusade—the mark of flames lick up from my pubic bone to just below my breasts, branding me as a mother for the rest of my days.

A twisted scar that splits my lower belly in two—the means of bringing my son and my daughter into this world, my son sucking desperately for air, my daughter stubbornly lodged under my ribcage.

These are the signs of my victory. The constant reminder of the two precious lives that are held—now and forever—in my own small and shaking hands.

Some women breeze through their pregnancies. They glow. They shine. They bloom with effervescence. I vomited. I grew so huge I could hardly move. My hips and pubic bone ached so badly the doctor ordered me to use a wheelchair when leaving the house. I developed a horrific rash that had me weeping with agony. The edema in my feet and legs was so bad that I could only force loose bedroom slippers on my feet. I gave birth while fighting a raging urinary tract infection.

In and out of the hospital during the last two months. Days of staring at the walls, unable to communicate with my weak Finnish, placed on a low calorie diet because the babies were so huge and I was so small, constantly hungry and struggling to get out of the narrow and hard hospital beds. Weeping silent tears, waiting the hours down, waiting for my wife to come and see me, breaking the monotony of my days, able to finally translate for me what the midwives had desperately tried to communicate to me in their stilted English.

Early labor that started at 33 weeks. The injections to stop it. The blood tests. The endless needles. The suffocation of the MRI to determine whether or not my pelvis, gaping open from pubis symphysis, would accommodate the babies. Chanting, "I'm not dead, I'm not dead," as I was shoved into the tiny enclosed grave, blasted with sound, my babies churning their terrified protests within.

Screaming and sobbing in the middle of the night in the week before the birth, unable to sleep, unable to breathe, a swollen abode of painful flesh. The desperate attempts of my wife to comfort me, to no avail.

The doctor took pity on me, finally, and scheduled a cesarean section on day one of my 36th week. No vaginal birth for me. My daughter transverse, lying horizontally deep in the womb. My pelvis, at risk of being damaged. I didn't care. It was their time. It was my time.

Laying in my hospital bed, scheduled for an 8:00 a.m. surgery. Another sleepless night. Trembling with the realization that this was it. My life was going to change. I wasn't ready. I was out of my carefully and lifelong cultivated control, taken over by hormones, by drugs, by pain.

My wife arriving in the morning, her face betraying her own sleepless night, despite her cheerful words. How her own large and capable hands shook as they held mine. Closing my eyes as she whispered to me how beautiful I was, how strong I was, how much she loved the babies and me. Her eyes haunted by fear and the memory of the losses she has already known. I try my own words of reassurance but they fall flat. We clutch each other's hands, holding on until they force us apart, me to the surgery room, her to change into scrubs and wait until called.

Being prepped, painted in wild pinks and yellows, antiseptics that would last for days on my skin. Hunching over and making "a back like an angry cat makes," being held as I could not keep the position myself. Trying not to cry out as the long snake of the epidural entered my spine. Listening to the instructions given to me by the gangly and efficient anesthesiologist, trying to focus on what I was to do. Looking in vain for my wife. The kindness of a nurse as she squeezed my hand and said, "Almost there, little mother." Wanting my wife so badly I forget to breathe. The oxygen mask knocking my glasses aside, raising a hand skewered with an IV to push them back into place. The agony of the catheter forced into my infected bladder disappearing as my lower half numbed itself. Hearing the doctors enter, but not seeing them due to the sheets draped between my breasts and belly. And finally, the smiling face of my wife, dressed head to toe in scrubs. "Don't I look cool," she asks, and I allow that she does. The look in her eyes as she wipes a stray splatter of blood off of my forehead. "You look so beautiful," she whispers, and I close my eyes as I feel a painless tug.

And then the cry, clogged with mucus and weak, but a cry. "Poika!" cries the doctor, and I know that my son has entered the world. The tears start, and drip down the oxygen mask. "There's Rasmus, do you hear?" my wife asks me, her face radiant. A moment later, another tug, and a stronger cry this time. "Tyttö," announces the birth of my daughter. I'm sobbing now, aching to see them. My wife is called over to look at them, and with a squeeze on my shoulder, she goes out of eyesight. I do not know then that my daughter is strangling on her own umbilical cord. They don't impart this news to the mother, helpless and gutted open on the table.

The nurse is there, smiling, and holding near my face a pair of the largest cheeks I have ever seen. "Your daughter," she says, and I raise my hand to rip the oxygen mask off of my face. I can smell her. I kiss her. She is the most exquisite thing I have ever seen. The nurse smiles and says, "We give her a bath with Äiti now." It does not occur to me until much later that she has used the Finnish term for Mother for my wife. A small victory, a great kindness.

Next up is my son, nose and mouth cleared of mucus. I am struck by his beauty—my mouth and the high Finnish cheekbones given to him by an anonymous man who donated his life seeds. They take him away and I am left to be repaired.

Drifting in and out of consciousness. Feeling sick at one point, the nurse adjusting my IV to keep me from vomiting. The background chatter of the doctors sewing me back together like a rag doll ripped apart at the seams. The smiling reassurances of the nurses. I am fading. I weep, thinking of my son's mouth and my daughter's cheeks. It's time to move me to the gurney, and my wife has reappeared. They will take me to recovery. My wife goes again to make phone calls, soothing anxiously awaiting Americans, waiting their middle of the night vigils in California. I sleep in recovery, an automatic blood pressure cuff squeezing my arm every five minutes. My wife is there again, and smiling, and telling me of speaking to my mother. I can not focus on her face, so I listen to the sound of her voice, her accent soothing me, the feel of her knuckles softly brushing my cheek.

I sleep.

I am in a hospital room. I do not remember getting there. My babies are laying together in an isolette. I stretch my arms out to them, and a midwife and my wife help me put them to my breasts. No milk yet, but I can feel their eager mouths on my skin. I cannot understand that they are mine. My chubby daughter, fine black hair cradling her head. My delicate son, black hair in whorls, tiny hands clutching at me. As I begin to fade, my wife gently puts them back, carefully tucking the covers over them. I watch her hands smoothing the silky blue blanket over their bodies.

I sleep.

We have survived. And at that moment, it is enough. Death can not have them. I will protect them. Their Äiti would die for them.

So I sleep.

As do they.

25

Maternal Web: La Luz de la Matriz

Jeannette Monsivais-Ruiter

I shifted my weight on the cream-colored futon as I sat in the waiting room at Maternidad la Luz, a midwifery clinic in El Paso. I continued reading from the book *Birthing from Within*; it said, "The day you give birth 300,000 women around the world will be giving birth, too." I had an image of an African woman giving birth in a pristine savanna landscape, of a Zapatista woman giving birth in the Chiapas jungle, and of a Tarahumara woman giving birth in the Sierra Tarahumara in Mexico. I told myself I would think of them when I was giving birth; I would try to imagine our powers united as we worked to bring our children into the world.

I lay the book on my very pregnant belly and thought about my great-grandmother who gave birth to six children, my grandmother who gave birth to eight children, and my mother who gave birth to three children; I wondered if they had known this comforting thought. I had a sense, though, that in the past women seemed to have an inherent knowledge that they were able to give birth. But more importantly, they did not seem to fear this natural process, at least not like I did. I was terrified, especially when people would point out how petite I am, or how painful it is to give birth without meds, not to mention the possible complications that could occur, such as the baby going into distress, in which case it would be recommended I have a c-section. All I wanted was to give birth the way my ancestors did, for my daughter to enter the world the way I did.

I heard my name called and smiled at Elenya, the midwifery student who would assist me in the birth of my baby.

Citas, or appointments, at the clinic usually lasted an hour and a half because they are very thorough. Checking my weight, urine, and blood pressure was merely the tip of the iceberg. At every *cita,* Elenya asked me what I ate the day before, as she checked off a list that confirmed I ate at least four things from each food group. She would ask if I was drinking my teas— raspberry tea to nourish the womb with calcium, and nettle tea for the extra iron; if I was taking my prenatal vitamins and drinking 8-12 glasses of water a day; if I was doing my yoga, walking, and doing my 100 daily kegels to improve the circulation and integrity of the perineum and to reduce the risk of tearing. After completing this checklist, Elenya would measure my stomach, feel the position of my baby, and listen to her heartbeat for the full five minutes.

I always looked forward to my *citas.* I felt like my questions and concerns were always heard. But more importantly, I felt connected to this community of women who have had children, who've guided and supported many women to bring forth their own children into the world, who educate other women about what is happening to their bodies throughout the pregnancy and during the labor. Oftentimes, I felt vulnerable when I was in public, but here in this community of warrior women, I felt empowered.

I dedicated one hour a day to practicing yoga. I stretched every limb, joint, and breathed deeply, visualizing the air traveling from my nose, past my throat, down my diaphragm, and finally to my sacrum. I'd sometimes rub my hands over my belly and feel my growing, baby girl. I would tell her these breaths I took were for her, and would be forever until they stopped.

I practiced the angle pose; the soles of my feet touched while my knees fell to the floor, and I raised my arms straight up on either side of my head. For three minutes, I breathed deeply in this pose. The first minute or two seemed easy, but my arms strained to stay in the air for the remaining time; I had to remind myself that I was building endurance for the labor. Filled with determination, I would close my eyes with the intent to let go of time, and to focus within.

Maternal Web: La Luz de la Matriz

After overcoming the moment of giving up with the will to keep going, I dreamed of traveling to an untouched part of the Chihuahua Desert where the valley between mountains of rock lay before me. I sat at the mouth of a cave and breathed deeply as I balanced the sun between my arms. It slowly descended behind the mountains in the background, and I felt the delicate contrast between the fire that warmed me from behind and the coolness that crept up from the shadows, which quickly spread across the Texas sage and ocotillo rooted in shifting sands. The cool air blew from the mountains, brushed over the branches of the palo verde, and rushed up my arms, shocking the veins stiff. I awoke to birds chirping outside the front door, wide open and connected to the sky, to the desert, to me, to my daughter.

They say there is something very special about having a girl, for she is born with all of the eggs she will ever have. As your daughter grows in your womb, therein lie your future grandchildren. I am descended from strong women, and strive to become like them; at one time I was a part of them, and they are part of me still. When my grandmother carried my mother, there was an intricate connectedness from my grandmother to my mother to me, seamlessly forming a part of one another in one space in time. And now as I held my daughter within me, I felt more connected to the women who came before me, and also linked to my future.

As my pregnancy settled into a seemingly permanent state, my due date arrived with not even the slightest hint of labor. I started to feel impatient for the big day, and I rejoiced over the mild cramps that arrived five days later. My husband David and I went over the supplies we'd be taking to the clinic: a case of water bottles, peanut butter, honey, bread, fruit, Gatorade, and clothes for my daughter and me.

The following morning I had sporadic cramps until two in the afternoon. We went to sleep that night disappointed that it was not yet time. I awoke at three in the morning to use the restroom; by then I was all too accustomed to taking nighttime bathroom breaks, but when I came back to bed, instead of nestling back into my warm space I was startled by soggy sheets. I nudged David's shoulder, urging him to wake up, and quickly called the clinic. The student on call told me to come in straight away, and asked if I was having contractions, but the contractions remained suspended as if waiting for a safe place to give birth.

As we drove through the dark, downtown streets of El Paso, I remembered the dream where I was sitting at the mouth of the cave; maybe I had mistaken the falling sun for the rising one. A pale yellow glow from the streetlights above guided us down the empty path we had traveled so many times before. I thought if I sat still enough the contractions would come, but instead I felt more water gush down from within me.

We arrived to the clinic; the hustle and bustle of the daytime *citas* had settled into a sleepy little nest with only light creaks coming from the hardwood floors. Elenya and Debbie reminded me that I would be participating in every aspect of the labor process, so it was very important that I rest for a couple of hours. But of course, I found I could not relax enough to fall asleep. My mind would race every time I closed my eyes, and I felt a great relief when Elenya finally came into our room at six o'clock to give me the castor oil to stimulate the contractions. Two hours later, as the sun came up, I felt the cramps emerge. Elenya encouraged me to walk around, squat, stretch, and made me a peanut butter and honey sandwich to give me energy to last through the labor. At this time, Debbie came off her shift, and Elizabeth, another staff midwife, took over.

Three hours after my contractions began, I felt as if my body was becoming less of my own—that I was no longer in control, but being carried by another force. Elenya reminded me to breathe deeply and evenly. I told her I needed to use the restroom, and she led me by the elbow. Normally this would have been uncomfortable, but I was starting to feel too much pain to worry about social graces. With each subsequent trip to the restroom, it became increasingly difficult to walk back to the birthing room. The last time I returned, I heard Elizabeth whisper to Elenya, "She's pushing."

I could feel the pain's intensity lessen when I pushed, and I hoped they would not ask me to stop. Elenya asked if she could check how dilated I was. She said it was fine if I didn't want to because they trusted that my body knew when it was time to push. I shook my head no, relieved that I had a choice.

Maternal Web: La Luz de la Matriz

Lying on my back, I felt the beads of sweat drip slowly down my face. My hair was disheveled. Individual strands tickled my face, but I was too concentrated to brush away the floating hairs. I tried to think about the African, Zapatista, and Tarahumara women, but I could not concentrate on anything other than my pushing. I held onto the wooden headboard, and pushed as long and hard as my body allowed, hoping I would not snap the headboard in half.

I closed my eyes after a contraction, and felt myself gliding past burning, desert sands shifting under the summer sun. They formed mini-sand dunes reaching past the mountains along the horizon. Then a breeze traveled across the sand transforming it into rippling water. I opened my eyes, and David placed a straw to my lips so I would drink.

There was a brief moment when I had fallen asleep, and I flew above a tunnel of oak trees and saw a tiny blue car swallowed by its archway, entering a cool, dark shade. I remained above this scene encased in a grey-blue mist, until the sharpness in my abdomen reminded me I was still in labor; I pushed until I thought my face would burst.

David and Elenya told me what a good job I was doing, and Elizabeth would place a Doppler to my belly to check my daughter's heartbeat.

After three hours of hard pushing, Elenya asked me if she could call in beginning students to witness my daughter's birth, and I saw my African, Zapatista, and Tarahumara sisters smile as they too neared the end of their rite/right of passage. I was sweaty and tired and pushed until Catherine's head came out, and two minutes later the rest of her followed. I was so relieved and proud that I did it, that I had not even noticed that one of Catherine's feet was still inside. Elenya quietly pointed it out to David, and he tugged out her tiny foot. It was as if she was holding on a bit longer to the matriarchal universe.

Elizabeth and Elenya cleared Catherine's nasal passages, wrapped her in a warm, white towel and a lavender hat with "La Luz", the light, written on its front. Elenya placed Catherine on my belly, and I cradled my past and my future comfortably upon my heart. After a lifetime of having her within me, and my body struggling to let her go, my heart leapt at the idea that this was just the beginning.

26

Shifts of Light:
The Transformative Nature of Birth

Karen Deaver

I am driven by the challenge of writing about how my son's birth transformed me, let me in on secrets I hadn't read or heard of in all my good-student preparations. My world, too, was rocked on that snow-covered January day, the one we'll celebrate with candles for my son. His birth accomplished a radical shift in my terrain—in my ability to cope, mentally, and in my perception of my body's strength and resilience. It took me from my comfortable, cerebral approach to life and thrust me into my earthly, primal, mortal self—a door that, once opened, continually reveals depths of light and shadow. Birth's result, life itself, grew me the fiercest visceral and emotional attachment possible, and with it layers of vulnerabilities and resolves I hadn't previously touched.

My expectations going in were abstract and naïve, even at the wise age of 37. They were, in a word, romantic. I imagined something orgasmic—a seamless transition from one state to another with a euphoric conclusion. My presumption was that the process, if done well, could be a linear production, and that, like an exam, the better prepared I was, the smoother the ride would be. And in some ways this was true. I studied with my husband the Bradley method of childbirth, asked questions of those that had gone before me, and watched videos of babies being gently coaxed into the world in hot tubs by peaceful women whose hair was soft and flowing. From my years as a dancer, I would rely on skills of body awareness and an ability to use images to calm myself, relax, and go with the flow. I believed in my birth team: husband, Steve; close friend Rachel; my mother, Julie; our midwife, Louise; and her assistant and our Bradley teacher, Barbara. With such a supportive and intelligent group as this, I had all I needed. And I was birthing at home, where I felt comfortable and safe.

Reality check: the prior knowledge that a mass, somewhere around eight pounds worth, was going to slowly move through my body toward its inevitably too small exit didn't register as any kind of guarantee of pain. Even though I knew it would hurt—maybe, I imagined, as my tonsillectomy had hurt, or my broken arm—I couldn't have imagined that kind of pain, one so all-consuming, focused, and brilliant that it was like a blinding light absorbing everything into itself: sound, sight, smell, taste. I couldn't have imagined having to hold on to those edges of my self that heretofore had solved most difficult situations by talking them through. In birth all is pre-language, the sounds of creation.

Though I was anxious in its anticipation, once begun, birth took me with it, in spite of my thorough preparation and the part of me that seems to be in control. Birth drowns "you" out with a predetermination that I have witnessed only once before, with death. It is nonnegotiable, intractable. It is, in the end, not rational, not controllable. With the first contraction I jettisoned these concepts, and along with it the neatly examined birth plan, methods of management, orchestrated civilities. I quickly realized that "I," my rational mind, was no match for this power. It was the animal part of me that would participate, the human that could listen for direction from within.

"It's like a volcano is erupting inside of me," another woman whispered during labor to my midwife. I deferred to it utterly. Even tenacious self-consciousness, the image of how I might "look" giving birth, was tossed, like so much else, to the back of my mind—back to a time long ago when I didn't notice so much, in childhood, or perhaps before. The people who had come to provide their arms and backs for me to lean on, who wiped my brow and remained peacefully present for 19 hours, dissolved into the very essence of their love for me. I knew only their eyes and their bones and muscles and that they never went away.

My labor was slow and persistent. It pushed along like a building river and lapped itself as was described in every textbook: first, ten minute contractions like small, consistent bites of memory. I was uncertain and wanted to focus on the possibility that this was labor, to assess my energy, all that had led to this place, and where I was going. I knew that something was up when I began to lose miserably at a game of Scrabble ... and I didn't care. I left the room to concentrate on the cramping that had begun, to breathe, lie down, and wear loose clothes. From then on, time was elastic: each minute lengthened, pulling each hour with it until there was just the constant pulsation of movement. Even as my body seemed to intensify, my mind became quieter, listening for the secret I was being told in a voice that became softer and softer.

I went to lie in the Jacuzzi. I had plans for this discomfort—the regular prodding that was not like burning but brief menstrual cramps. More like a swarm of worker bees hell bent on deconstructing a hive. Five hours into it, at 2 a.m., with contractions four minutes apart, we called for my mother, and she, too, became part of the rhythm of hand holding and kind, expectant eyes. Our midwife, Louise, was called and arrived an hour later, awake, professional, hovering on the outside perimeter of my now completely internal world, one where sound and touch and smell, sucked into this force of nature like cows into a tornado, had become grossly magnified and near intolerable. Steve wanted to massage me, but each touch was an invasion. Music or chatting was deeply disturbing. I fell inward, to a place of extreme focus, but one without thought, sometimes so peaceful, moaning to myself during each rise and drifting away, inside, with each fall. I was aware of time only in its shifts of light and darkness rising and descending around us. I felt burrowed in to last as long as birth would, and I screened out any but the reverential or directive voices and hands of the team nearby.

Louise brought with her the knowledge of these secrets, and of the raw physiology driving them, that Steve and I faithfully depended upon. Her ability and care were all reassurance, her powerful body and voice calm but decisive. Her reasonableness made me want to scream, to cry out that this experience was not reasonable. Though she asked me to focus on the future, on the baby, I couldn't. There was too much else to get through me.

192

Shifts of Light

Transition came after 18 hours had disappeared like a collapsed star into the tight-knit space we occupied. I was in water, fighting with my reasonable, deal-making self, who had reappeared in one last attempt to ease pain: If I just lie here and breathe, all will be still. I hoped to stall the inevitable, but my body knew that there was only one way out. "Move through it," Louise whispered repeatedly; relax the undersides of your thighs; try standing up. Stand up? I thought. With gravity comes more pain comes baby.

It all made sense, but still, still. The body fights with the mind: Stay calm, it will go away. Float through it, find its pleasure; sing the moaning tide through to the other side. The baby, the life on its own course, pushing forward, not knowing air from amniotic fluid, would come despite what I thought. So I stood and sang and saw that the quotidian calm and empathy in the faces around me contradicted my sense that something was dreadfully wrong. The baby's heartbeat was steady, strong; a colt galloping to the finish. All was normal—welcome to the sisterhood.

In the bedroom, I grabbed hold of a bedpost and visualized one good squat and the crowning push, all with great ease and beauty, as South American women did it—at least on videos—quietly, expectantly, a smile on their lips. After several monumental pushes using a force and determination that yielded a growling, jugular sound more animal than human, I sat, and Louise placed my hand on the point of our baby's head. (*It's coming, it's coming!*). Its wet firmness receded with the contraction, taking with it a piece of me I wasn't sure I could recover the next time around. The uncertainty made me more determined, and at Louise's suggestion I moved again, businesslike, up on to the bed, where I held my legs back and pushed and howled and progressed.

50 minutes of pushing became the one push that released my baby's head through the opening of my body, which now felt more like a strip mine than a private garden. (Steve would later tenderly tell me that he hadn't realized that that delicate flower was so tough). Time began to unwind, rushing back into the space as though a vacuum seal had been broken: light filled the room even on the grayest of January days, air filled my lungs. The world seemed to reclaim its usual proportions, and my consciousness of it returned to record every detail. With

another push, our baby's body was out and I was reaching downward in one fell swoop, a bird capturing its young as it falls, scripted to fly. He had mass, earthiness. He was mine: blue, wet, heavy, warm. Mine. Ours. The world's. I seemed to recognize him, our son, who was like an old friend in my arms. The placenta, like a separate yet equal twin, released itself from my insides with another push and tug, and with its exit there came the greatest relief of all. We all breathed together the sweet air as we rubbed blue to pink and stared.

The days that followed were surreal; they overflowed with extremes of emotion brought on by a tango of hormones. I was in ecstasy of life's generosity one moment and in wretched awareness of its tenuousness the other. My mind made repeated efforts to comprehend the physical violence my body had just endured. What lay beneath my chin seemed a foreign territory, discarded, bloodied, and stitched. I was raw, even though the actual damage was slight: a very small labial tear that required one stitch. Recovery, of course, comes simultaneously with the demands of a nursing, crying newborn, and there are no magical skills that appear for coping with the immediate and dramatic changes. I learned to be grateful for the gifts that came along with the challenges. The energy my son and I were exchanging at the breast created a unique rhythm quite apart from the measured, predictable days of yore. I alternately looked into his new eyes for answers and for secrets. *I will remember this day for him,* I vowed. *He will always know how he came, and how his mother came, too.* A new vessel opened in my heart that day, a very tough one that remains, like my birth howls, without words.

27

Sheila's Vine

Tania Pryputniewicz

Ghost

I used to read their bodies as they sauntered in. Without the weight of names or the past, it's all in the posture. There's always one student in the class I'm teaching whose story I know like my own.

That summer, it was Sheila, a girl with a quarter inch halo of hair, a leather choker around her neck, and a thin blue skirt that floated clear of her slim thighs. She wafted into her seat and folded her legs, revealing a winding vine tattoo around her ankle. Her life's dream, she told my English class during introductions, was to become a midwife. Through her journal entries, which she bordered with thick black vine and leaf doodles, I learned she had a close friend who was pregnant. Sheila was looking forward to witnessing the birth as the first step of many towards her dream of midwifery. I also learned her parents had recently divorced; she was living in the mildewed basement, choosing it for its placement as the room furthest from her new stepfather.

I remember when my parents first divorced, night after night my little sister cried herself to sleep. We shared a room by the front steps where the lion gold of the porch light filtered through the curtains. Over the incessant sound of my father playing piano, we'd listen for my mother's car until sleep overcame us. On weekends, we'd visit the farmer's market, gravitating towards the sunflowers in buckets and the baskets of fist sized geodes I mistook for meteorites. I held them in my palms, crystal innards to the sky. I recognized that same rawness, something broken open, in Sheila.

Both in journal entries and class discussions, Sheila was an advocate for the homeless. She personally knew one of the authors of an essay we read about people who collected anything salvageable out of dumpsters, from clothing to food. I often chose example passages from her writing to share with the class, due to her strong and moving use of language. During office visits, she confided her love for her boyfriend, a steadying force against a burgeoning feeling of disconnection with her mother.

Sheila chose to write her final paper on labor and delivery, concluding with a paragraph on the upcoming birth she'd be attending over the summer break. She was one of two "A" students in the class. "I can't wait for the birth of this baby," she told me during our last conversation.

"I want to hear how it goes," I said, not a mother yet myself, still a single community college instructor. I urged Sheila to visit and consider taking a creative writing class with me in the future. A week later, the head of the department called to tell me Sheila had committed suicide; she'd argued with her boyfriend and had suffered a relapse with heroin usage. It was the first I'd heard of her addiction.

I went straight to my shelf and took down the folder of final papers. I let them fall to the floor, searching for Sheila's. There was her name, and on the title page, the familiar vines and leaves, delicate as one of those intricate ink tattoos you see running up the arms of girls from India, embroidered across the backs of their hands to trail gracefully up each arm. I held the essay in my hand.

Something left my heart, small as a blossom pulled from an apple tree by a drop of rain.

Then it was back: that she'd done it. I pulled myself to the living room and curled up in my reading chair, knees to chest, and waited for dusk.

There was nowhere to go but back in time. To the vortex of the one moment I wondered whether it was worth it to live or not. When I finally realized my parents' divorce was real, I spent the night on the sand down by the river. Before the sun came up, I etched a line across my wrist with a piece of glass. But before I could draw blood, my sister's voice came calling me through the trees.

Sheila's Vine

The sound of her voice was so real, I stood up and looked for her behind me, but no one was there, just the dawn on its way. I thought, *I would never want to find my sister dead, so I will never put her in that position.* And I climbed the cold sandy path back through the trees to my house. My eighth grade teacher pulled me aside that week and offered to take me into her home. My parents refused the invitation, but the fact that she offered mattered deeply and I always remembered that act of love.

At Sheila's service, inside the funeral home, the family arranged a display in a semi circle at the front of the room, like an altar at one of those places where the Virgin Mary had been sighted. Candles on multi-leveled tiers flickered behind works of Sheila's art on easels, buried in dozens of bouquets of red, white and yellow roses. The pastor read from a letter Sheila had left for her preteen sister and young brother in which she apologized, telling them how much she loved them. Seeing Sheila's little sister cry, and her young brother sitting so stiffly and quietly on the edge of his chair, I had to leave the room.

The sky was a deep indigo blue. Across the street, an elementary school parking lot was filling for an event. Car doors slammed over the din of the voices of children and parents. The first few stars of the night poked through, oddly bright. Closer. Like the sky had been torn.

What about the rest of us on Earth? I asked Sheila, the sky.

I'd quelled the suicidal impulse in myself that day on the riverbank.

But there are many ways of dying. There was something about the two halves of the whole—mother, father, rejecting one another—and moving in to my stepfather's home, where the chairs and chandeliers and beds belonged to him. And an overwhelming urge to run. So one morning when I was 14, I put on my blue jogging shorts. And ran down the street. A boy, 19, a friend of a friend who lived two blocks over, came out of his house. Orange curtains with dark brown tulips covered the windows. A sink of unwashed dishes. Lemon dish soap and rotting meat. A glass jug of vodka.

Later that afternoon, I hid in my stepfather's bathroom, locking myself in, panicking at the sight of the blood on my thighs. My 13-year-old brother came to the other side of the door and begged me to let him in. He wanted to find and fight the boy who had done this. But I swore him to secrecy, and after that he made himself scarce; by the end of that month, he moved out of my stepfather's home to live with our father again.

It took years for me to understand it wasn't my fault for entering the boy's house or for taking a drink. I remember the leader of a survivor's group in college explaining the whole timeline of healing to me, back when she first interviewed me for the group. She drew a line on a sheet of paper, with an x, dead center, marking the incident.

Where do you think you are now? She asked me, and I'd drawn an x at the farthest edge of the paper.

That's what you think, she said, smiling, *but actually you are here,* and she'd put an x right beside the first one. That had enraged me, to think something that happened ten years ago could still be staining my life now. But the survivor's group did help me to see that there were two of us in the room, and that one of us chose to take advantage, and one of us did not.

The night of Sheila's funeral, I woke at three a.m. In the gray grainy air of my bedroom, dark green leaves and vines clung and whirled across the lip of my mattress. The vines roped along my pillow, tendrils reaching for my face.

Grief rippled through my body.

"Hi girl," I said gently.

For a long moment, I sat in Sheila's presence. I felt the same core questions swirling up out of her—her search for a place she could call her own. I wanted to protect her from the truth: that she no longer had a body through which to move about in this world. But she seemed to know she was transient, with but a few seconds to hold shape. And yet she hesitated.

"Go back, Sheila," I said at last. "It's alright, go back..."

And slowly the vines turned inchworm green, then luminescent blonde, then white, like sunlight striking corn. The air cleared and I began my own disintegration into the field of dreams, comforted by the awareness that the soul keeps its longings between incarnations.

Midwife

Seven years later, when I found myself pregnant for the second time, and having had a first birth experience laced with hospital interventions (breaking of my water, pitocin to speed contractions, epidural to withstand the shock and force of pitocin-induced contractions, threat of the 24-hour timeline towards a c-section), I decided to look into hiring a midwife, remembering Sheila's passion for the role, associating "midwife" with an inexhaustible list of nurturing qualities. My husband Mark and I found a private birth facility where the intake woman welcomed us, commenting, "You're our perfect candidate—a woman whose first birth experience in a hospital was less than desirable, a woman who is clear about what she wants."

We believed her when she said, "Even if you have complications and end up at the hospital, you're still guaranteed our expert care, and your birth plan will be followed." And we believed the pages of personal intake information would be read and taken into consideration—especially the answer to the question: Is there anything specifically in your past you wish us to know about so we can better serve you?

I mulled over the intake form, deciding to be honest: I had some residual feelings of vulnerability and fear about giving birth due to the childhood rape. During my first birth experience, people I had not invited came against my previously stated wishes and stayed in the birth room, stirring up feelings of violation. I was reassured that this time around, I would have complete control over who was in the room.

After a facility tour and a brief introduction to the three midwives on staff, the intake secretary explained we'd see all three midwives during the course of my pregnancy, and while I was free to choose one of them as my primary caregiver, they couldn't promise which of the three would be available for the actual birth. I remember having a good feeling about two of them; one, red-haired and tall, seemed hurried and distant, but I passed over it in my joy to have found an alternative setting with its warm pastel walls, couches with velvet pillows, framed paintings, bouquets of flowers, full kitchen. We were told we could look forward to positive affirmations from the midwives during my labor (I could write these myself ahead of time) and sensitive care.

Sensitive care included time with their birth counselor debriefing from the first birth, a doula service (which provides you with a private birth helper, akin to a labor coach), and a birth mandala workshop (meditation followed by time to create one's own mandala, each spiraling out from a ten centimeter diameter circle—that painstaking distance one's cervix needs to dilate). We used and enjoyed all three of the services. Our doula was a nursing student who made herself entirely available to us, leaving her own three-year-old son home with his father during the night of the birth.

After my third session with the birth counselor, I worked up the courage to discuss presences I'd been sensing and seeing following Sheila's suicide. Over the years I'd learned to keep things to myself—one friend had said to me, "You know, they have medication for that—go see a psychiatrist." So I played it safe, describing an innocuous encounter from one drowsy afternoon: upon waking from a nap, I saw three babies floating near the bedroom wall, downy curls on their heads, plump mottled cheeks touching.

"Which one of you will it be?" I thought at the time, amused by the incoming souls vying for the pregnancy.

But I was more disturbed by the strange man and his teenage son at the foot of my bed, and later, the tall woman in a cloak hovering outside my closet doors. With the birth counselor's help, I understood some of it; I accepted the woman as a guardian, and connected her to the college rape survivor's group. I had a room-mate then who would hold me and make hot milk for me when I'd wake from nightmares of being chased by men, of falling only to be ripped in half. Dreams of flying so fast, I'd melt at the core.

One of those 2 a.m. nights, my roommate took me by starlight down the paved bike path, out past the freshman dormitories, past the bus barn to the open fields, where the tractors had trawled up the earth in heart-sized chunks. She picked up a clod and gave it to me. Then she picked up one of her own. There's nothing like the thwack they made hitting the ground, bursting open, and the smell of damp earth. We covered 25 yards of the bike path with busted clods. I went home with the scent of onion bulbs on my palms and slept without dream for the rest of the night.

Through the birth counseling sessions, I became less afraid of what I was seeing. I decided to include the guardian in my birth mandala. I drew my husband and me, bordering the focal cervix using soft red and blue colored pencils. Gathering around the rest of the cervix, I penciled in my father, doula, midwife, and a few extra bodies representing invisible helpers. I planned to bring the finished artwork to the birth facility and tape it to the mirror of my room.

13 days after my due date, we discovered by ultrasound that I had low amniotic fluid. My husband and I had counted on having a water birth, deposit on file, all set to use the birth tub at the facility. But the staff informed me that the low amniotic fluid level meant that I'd have to go to the hospital unless I could get myself into labor by the following morning. I was reminded I'd still have one of the midwives attending the birth itself, just up at the hospital instead of at the facility. My husband and I went down the list of 13 items on the "get yourself into labor" list, everything from strenuous hiking to vigorous sex to drinking large amounts of castor oil, to no avail. I spent much of the night in the bathroom, contraction free as the sun rose.

At 8:00 a.m., we headed for the hospital. Unfortunately, I'd written an incriminating birth plan that included what my husband and I felt was wrong with the hospital's approach at the birth of our first child. That very birth plan now was being transferred from the birth facility to the hospital for my midwife and the hospital staff to share. As I sat propped up in bed, dressed in my blue and white backless smock, I wondered which of the midwives would deliver my son.

A nurse inserted a pill against my cervix to help it dilate. I walked the hospital grounds for the next four hours as mild contractions set in. I was given a second pill, and by 4:00 p.m., the contractions grew strong enough so I had to pause on the fire-escape stairs to wait out the contractions (now spaced roughly 15 minutes apart). Encouraged to be progressing, I felt calm and relaxed about going into harder labor on my body's terms. Near the hospital entrance, I spotted a familiar figure approaching—red pony-tail visible over her fleece vest. She passed me at a good clip, pausing just long enough to tell me she'd be in to check my cervix shortly.

I expected her to ask how I thought things were going. Instead, she walked into the room and knelt down on the bed. "Let's check you," she said, pushing my knees apart and proceeding to insert her hand into my body so hard, my head hit the bedboard, her knuckles forcing past the folds of my skin. After one more jab to ascertain dilation, she withdrew her wrist, stood up and said, "Your cervix is still exactly the same. You're not dilating. Let's get the pitocin going." She turned and left.

Mark said, "Jesus, is that how those exams always go?"

"What..." I said, starting to cry, "was *that*?"

The bruises lasted for several weeks, still visible when the home visiting nurse came to check up on the stitches and the breastfeeding.

Our doula stepped in from the hallway—having missed the exchange entirely. When I told her what happened, she took me by the shoulders and said, "Your baby needs you. Put this behind you—we have to go on. You need the midwife to get through the birth." I fought to remain calm.

The nurse returned and hooked me up to the pitocin drip. "Can I still walk?" I asked.

"You can stand," she said, "but it's too much for you to wheel this around with you." She added, "Could you keep it down? Try and scream through your contractions with a lower voice."

I had endured pitocin from the first birth and was keenly aware of what I was about to face. From 5:00 to 7:00 p.m., I withstood the slamming contractions, holding onto my husband's shoulders, our doula rubbing my lower back. The midwife rechecked me at 7:00, told me I was dilated now to five centimeters, and left. The nurse popped in and reported, "Your midwife says we're turning up the pitocin. She wants you to have good hard labor for the next hour."

"Then give me an epidural," I said, between contractions.

Now the midwife came on board with the birth plan: she reappeared in the doorway long enough to remind me, "You told us you wanted a drug-free birth. I want you to reconsider. Do you really want an epidural?"

"Yes, she does," my husband said firmly.

When the anesthesiologist arrived, the nurse who had earlier asked me to be quiet stopped with the administration of an IV long enough to wipe the tears off my face. As the epidural kicked in, I felt a sense of peace and rightness. In charge of the birth again.

Shortly, they lost my baby's heartbeat. The room filled with nurses. I looked up into the bright lights over the bed and succumbed to fears of the worst: c-section, loss of my child. I glanced at my birth mandala, with its circle of beings floating around the red/blue swirl of cervix, and prayed for help. When they found the heartbeat, it was very slow. The nurse pulled an oxygen mask down over my face. As the cool air sheathed my nose and lips, I turned and watched the monitor: the miniature bouncing heart representing my baby's life. Over the next hour, he stabilized. We waited for the upped pitocin to do its work.

At three minutes to midnight, I pushed my son out. The epidural had backed off some and I could feel my legs and thighs, the strength of my pushes. I threw up just after; my body shook for an hour after he was born, a good shaking. They put my son on my belly, still attached to his cord. He nursed for a few minutes before they cut the cord. I watched his fist gripping the side of the mini-gurney under the heat lamp as they measured him.

"You're bruised," the midwife said curtly, mystified, as she stitched up my third degree tear. I didn't respond, focusing on my son instead, reveling in that first glance of knowing and longing—his dark blue birth-wet eyes locked on mine. When I could stand to let him go, I handed him to my father, who was in the delivery room for those 15 minutes of pushing. I called my mother (who I'd chosen to stay with my two-year-old daughter for the night of the birth). Hearing Mom's voice, I cried, and said, "He's here, and we're all ok."

I'll always be grateful he's here, and healthy. But the next morning, I did report to the visiting midwife the facility had sent to check on us that I was disturbed by what happened during my labor.

"Your son was the fifth delivery for us that day," she apologized, adding that my midwife was busy rushing from the facility to the hospital, as three of her expectant mothers were at the hospital with complications. "Why don't you wait and see how you feel, and when you come in for your two month checkup, if you still feel upset, you can talk directly to her about it."

I tried to stay in the moment, enjoying my infant, and loved how my daughter came to the room and put lotion on her new brother's arms. I loved my first cup of coffee that morning, and being able to put eggs into a stomach that now had room to digest them. In my first journal entry, three weeks after my son was born, I wrote:

What you don't expect before you have your second child is how much you love and miss your firstborn even living side by side with them, under the raging intensity of the needs of your infant second born. It's all welcome and I'm in the wide-eyed realization stage that I chose this and want to open my arms to it instead of curling up in defeat, as I'm in the third week of healing. Week one every cell hurt and I was bleeding internally as well as emotionally from the incident with the midwife—some kind of ex-enemy from a former lifetime...Mark lamenting all the work we did to get over having an extra person in the room at the first birth, and now this. Rather than let it fester, I wrote the midwife a letter. What she did reopens the childhood wound, but now I'm an adult--I can take action, even if after the fact.

A month after I mailed my letter to the birth facility, I received an apology note from the midwife with an invitation for me to come in and see her. Both she and the director of the facility attributed the bruising to the birth itself, denying it could have to do with any excessive force on the part of the midwife during the pelvic exam. They pointed out if I hadn't had an attending midwife, I probably would've been forced to have a c-section.

I spoke one last time to their birth counselor, but found myself unable to trust her by association. I told her what had happened over the phone, and got the classic well-meaning response, "This is a great opportunity for you to confront this, and it would be healing for you when you are ready to come in and talk to your midwife in person."

I chose not to see the midwife and gave the hospital a copy of my letter, asking that they keep it on file in hopes of protecting other birthing mothers who might be assigned to the midwife. Despite her apology, I couldn't bring myself to understand how she could be forceful enough to bruise and not know it. I grieved in the middle of the night, when my son's tug at the breast shot post-partum pains through the three layers of stitches. I'd try to slough off the confused feelings of braided sorrow and shame.

Later, I played back the whole string of events with the midwife, and unearthed two separate instances where I overrode my intuition.

The first time I went to the birth facility for my interview, I held the door open for a woman entering the building behind me. Her long silver hair was swept back from her face with a Celtic knot, and she carried an overflowing box of apples. As she set them down in the foyer with a "take me" note, I let myself fantasize she was one of the midwives. Something in her black natural fiber pants, generously soft figure, rosy cheeks, and careful handling of the apples made me relax instantly, and I thought, *Now, there's a woman I would trust to deliver my child.*

During that first tour with my husband, I learned I was right: she was one of three midwives, and her name was Martha. I was happy for a number of my prenatal visits when luck was with me and I "got" Martha. But somewhere during the third trimester, I began to see a lot of the midwife who eventually delivered my son. During one exam, I remember her trying to talk me out of a routine test Martha had recommended. I thought it odd she should argue so vehemently against Martha's suggestion, and did have the brief thought, *I better end up with Martha.* But as I recounted my funny feelings to my husband later that afternoon, I said, "But I'm probably being a hormonal pregnant woman. I should trust all three midwives."

The second time I had a chance to listen to my intuition was at the mandala workshop. There were six of us mothers, sitting around drinking prenatal tea and eating split pea soup in the birth therapist's home, drawing our cervix mandalas. The pregnant woman to my left was nursing a cold and I was irritated as my due date was less than a week away. The only other second-time mom, across from me on a purple pillow, was also using the birth facility for her delivery, and she looked right at me and said, "If you are having any doubts whatsoever about any of the midwives, make sure you ask for who you want."

I had a twinge in the gut, but I thought, *How could I at this late stage request one particular midwife without hurting the other two midwives' feelings?* Again I discounted my intuition. I ended up with the midwife I had doubts about.

I was given a relatively mild lesson about the cost of ignoring intuition: I didn't die at the midwife's hands, nor did my child. But I will listen more closely from now on, call the loved ones who appear in distressing dreams, change my plans for the day if I need to, pay attention to the people in my environment. I need to use that good radar (that we're all born with) and pass the skill on to my daughter and the son who survived, firsthand, the side-effects of my poor choice of caregiver during his descent towards the birth canal.

As for the midwife, maybe she had a bad day, hurrying from birth job to birth job; maybe she was just careless for that one pelvic exam and it was an isolated incident. Now that five years have passed since the birth of my son, I forgive her. What woman of today arrives where she is without some kind of trauma? But my prayer remains the same: that my letter make her pause to think about the access she has to touch women who are giving birth and not take for granted the trust placed in her. And for myself, that my grief over her trespass continue to fade from darkness to white, and disappear from my life, like Sheila's vine.

Seer

On the heels of my son's birth, the presences continued visiting: a turn of the century woman in a black cloak, then a man in a hat, urging me out of my blue grief, propelling me to seek out a consultation with a psychic to help me sort out what I was experiencing.

The psychic was a young mother herself. She told me that in a former life I bled to death at the hands of someone in England—one of those uterus mangling maniacs—and that I somehow hooked up with the midwife in this lifetime as a way to release emotion residing in the womb, stuck in my soul's remembering. That this milder incident with the midwife had struck a much deeper chord with an assault in which I died, thus explaining heightened feelings in this life. She suggested I was ready to move the old blockage out of my body, and crossing paths with the midwife was perhaps one way my soul chose to release the energy.

This explanation felt a little "out there," even for me—but I was ultimately grateful it prompted me to write a letter in which I explicitly confronted the midwife, something I'd not had the guidance or strength to do as a teen. Further, the psychic taught me I could have control over the visiting presences; I could decide if I wanted to be approached, suggesting I was unwittingly "open" psychically. I haven't determined if the presences are dream projections, entities, or leftover imprints from another time, but I asked that they stop for now and they have.

One gift the midwife gave me was a clear understanding of trespass. Her behavior was so clearly outrageous to me (and my husband) that I realized it had little to do with me. (Which means the same is true of the childhood incident— no need to blame myself for the actions of another person.) Past lives aside, I wish to be as present as possible for each day I am in my children's lives. I don't think I'm meant to believe I caused the chain of events with the midwife but I can seek to understand them in a way that makes me want to wake up in the morning. How we handle what happens to us can make the difference between life and death, as I learned from my talented but confused student, Sheila.

I was not a mother, back when I ran into Sheila's mother a year after the funeral.

I was still teaching then, and working part time for a real-estate agent who coincidentally was representing one of the family's properties. I had to deliver documents to Sheila's mother. I told the agent I didn't think it was appropriate I go, but he handed the folder to me and pointed to the door.

"You're Sheila's teacher, aren't you?" Sheila's mother said when I walked in. "How are you? Please, don't feel strange. Come talk to me. I'd love to show you some of her drawings sometime." She hugged me fiercely, brought me a cup of tea, motioned for me to set the documents down. Said nothing about the tears welling up in her eyes, just adjusted her glasses and left her other hand on my back.

"Hardest part for me, about her artwork," her mother continued, "is how obsessed she seemed with death."

This seemed so unlike the Sheila I had come to know. I remembered how alone Sheila felt, her sense of abandonment in the wake of her parents' divorce. I didn't blame Sheila's mother for the suicide, not exactly, but at the time I didn't have a reference point for the complexities of being a mother.

"I just want Sheila back," was the last thing she said to me before I walked out the door.

Now that I am a mother, and I think back to that moment in time with Sheila's mother, I am reminded of the chapter in *The Prophet* by Kahlil Gibran, in which he addresses the subject of children: *You may house their bodies but not their souls, For their souls dwell in the house of tomorrow, which you cannot visit, not even in your dreams.*

And after all my experiences with sensing presences, I would say to Sheila's mother, *But you can. You can visit her in dream. And she, you.*

28

On the Day You Were Born, the Angels Got Together

Ashini J. Desai

My husband's Aunt Sudha calls him her "baby." After all, as his father's youngest sister, she was present at the birth and held him when he was ten minutes old. And, she will be sure to tell everyone that within the first 15 minutes of acquaintance. At her son's wedding, she first introduced the bride and groom individually to the guests, and then her other "baby" and his new wife.

So it should not have come as a surprise when she said she wanted to be present at the birth of our first child. Initially, my husband Sandeep and I disregarded her declaration. She lived in Niagara Falls, Canada, at least eight hours from our home in Philadelphia. If I went into labor, she could not come down so quickly. Besides, having a houseguest when we were bringing home a new baby seemed like unnecessary stress. I had already decided that my mother, my sister Shivani and Sandeep would be present at the birth. No one else needed to be there. Moreover, per our Indian family tradition, I would be staying at my parents' home for a few weeks after the delivery; this would allow me to recover and focus on the baby without household obligations.

During the weeks leading to the due date, we received desperate phone calls from Aunt Sudha's three children.

"We tried to stop her but we can't."

"I told her, 'They don't need you there,' but she refuses to listen. I'm so sorry."

My husband and I finally conceded when she announced that she had bought her bus tickets and notified her work of her pending absence. We offered her a plane ticket at least, but she refused. Aunt Sudha has been an independent single mother for more than 20 years, always made her own way, and is an eccentric artist. I recognized the vein of stubbornness that runs through the family.

On my due date of February 5th, there was a sudden snowstorm dropping 14 inches of snow. I feared being the woman on the news who gave birth in a snow-plow. Thankfully, the baby had no intentions of coming. However, a week later, I was wondering if she was waiting for spring. Finally, I was going to be induced and the nurse asked if I liked Tuesday or Wednesday better. Definitely Wednesday. It was Valentine's Day.

We called our families and let them know of the induction. My parents were in New Jersey, and ready to hop on the Turnpike to Pennsylvania. My mother put in her request for personal time. My sister had flown to California on a job interview and would be taking the red-eye back on Wednesday. She was begging me to hold off delivering until she returned.

Aunt Sudha left Monday night from Niagara Falls and arrived Tuesday morning. She had changed buses every hour and a half, taking a total of six buses. She was a remarkable sight. Her shock of salt and peppery hair declares she's in her fifties. Her round face has soft wrinkles, but her laughter is youthful. She was standing at the bus station and her five-foot frame was overloaded with shopping bags. The majority of bags were gifts she had created for the baby; she planned to present them at the right moment. She had also thrown in a few changes of rumpled clothes. When she remembered, she would pull her hair back in a clip, though strands would weave themselves out of it.

On Tuesday evening, Sandeep, Aunt Sudha, and I went to the hospital to prepare for Wednesday's induction. We thought it would be a brief process and we would be done quickly. However, they wanted to monitor the baby's heart since it moved around so much. Sandeep, a typical Type A personality, restlessly paced the room and frequently visited the nurses' station, asking how much longer. His anxiety reflected back to me, as I lay there hooked to the fetal monitors, feeling quite large and nervous. Aunt Sudha kept rubbing my feet, as if to rub away the stress of the moment. She forced Sandeep to sit down and relax.

"This is not about you!" she scolded.

Sandeep surrendered and I was relieved she was there. A nurse named Lisa came on duty and lightened the mood with stories and light banter. We felt more relaxed in her presence and Lisa said she hoped to see us tomorrow when the baby was born. We were leaving two and a half hours after our arrival.

That night, I did my backstretches leaning on the kitchen counter, trying to relieve the pain. My husband looked at me sympathetically. I felt contractions at 10:00 p.m. and then again at 10:30 p.m. We sat in bed with our paper handy to track the contractions. However, we fell asleep until the next one occurred at 1:00. Aunt Sudha had warned us that if my water broke during the night, our new king-size mattress would be ruined. Sandeep pulled out an old plastic shower curtain and had me sleep atop that. I didn't mind since I was so uncomfortable and did not plan to sleep anyway.

We all rose at 5:00 a.m. and took warm showers. I called the hospital at 6:30 and they could see me in an hour. Sandeep donned his favorite sweat suit and I wore my now well-worn maternity clothes. Aunt Sudha snapped pictures of us preparing to leave.

"One last time with the big belly!" she cheered. We forced nervous smiles for posterity.

It was funny to enter as a normal person, and then suddenly be instructed to wear the hospital gown and lie in bed like an invalid. The good thing about a labor induction was that it was scheduled. This was the first grandchild in our family, so excitement was at a height. My mother and Shivani arrived promptly at 8 a.m. Shivani was still wearing her travel clothes: a black cardigan with a fluffy fur collar, black pants, and mules. I told her that only on *Sex and the City* did anyone wear heels in the delivery room. She was too jet-lagged to respond. My mother had packed a tote bag with books and snacks for everyone. For me, she had packed traditional foods that new mothers should eat. There were some herbs for teas to promote lactation, including poppy seeds and fenugreek. She had prepared other delicacies rich in milk, butter and sugar, which would help replenish the body of lost nutrients. They were topped with other special seeds and spices. I smelled these foods and just pushed them away. I was supposed to eat and drink that for the next few months?

By 9:00 a.m., they started the I.V. with pitocin. Sandeep actually left the room because he wasn't sure if he could watch the IV tube be inserted. We all wondered if it was wise for him even to think about the birth. My mother approached the nurse and politely asked, "How long will it take for the baby to come now?"

The nurse laughed. "Who knows? It can happen immediately or for hours. We'll just wait and see!" We all looked a bit confused. In a world of structure and schedules, it seemed odd to have such uncertainty.

Around 9:30 a.m., a resident asked if it would be all right if medical students came to review obstetrics. *This is a teaching hospital, just like on* ER, I told myself. I agreed and in walked five attractive young men. I could swear one was Matt Damon and I preened my hair. I wanted to tell them, "I'm normally not this pregnant."

The resident told them how to poke and feel for the head of the baby, and she would demonstrate first. I lay there with my big belly protruding and tried to tuck my blanket around to preserve a shred of modesty. Each shy student first said "Hi" to me and then poked my belly. One student was so nervous he barely poked me, and I wanted to take his hand and show him how to do it. In between two students at the foot of the bed appeared Aunt Sudha with her camera.

"No pictures!" I cried.

"Oh, don't worry. I'm not getting you," she replied. "I'm getting all the good looking doctors!" The guys blushed for the camera.

"After her, if anyone wants to feel me, you can!" she offered enthusiastically. The room just laughed. I decided I would give up now.

I pulled out my John Edwards relaxation tape and headphones, and tried to focus my "mind's eye" on soothing colors. I had listened to this tape a lot during my pregnancy and it would often put me to sleep. I thought this would be perfect, since I never got around to the birth hypnotherapy.

Throughout the day while I labored, Shivani sat with me and asked if the contractions really did hurt. I tried to describe every painful moment. We watched the monitor and I felt every wave. I tried to listen to John Edwards, but he really started to annoy me. I could care less about his stupid colors. I took off my headphones and threw it on the side table. My sister stumbled across the room in her state of jet lag and I yelled at her to get over it. She was hurt and just walked out.

In the meantime, Aunt Sudha chatted with my mom to distract her. My mom was nervous and did not know what to expect, especially seeing her daughter go through the pain. Periodically, Aunt Sudha would come to me and give a fabulous foot rub and some comforting words. The best part was that she was support for my husband. We all talk about support for the mother, but I never thought the fathers would need support too. When I needed to have the epidural, Sandeep hesitated. He wasn't sure if he could be there, given his aversion to needles. She told him he must go and support me. I never found out what she said to him, but it was a good pep talk.

Throughout the procedure, Sandeep held my hand and looked at my face as the anesthesiologist did his work. The doctor's professionalism made the epidural go well. He made small talk about children to relax us a little. Then he walked us through the procedure so I could prepare myself. It made the experience much better than I feared.

However, immediately after the epidural was administered, they noticed the heart rate of the baby had descended. Everyone panicked. I heard the word "c-section" being thrown around. Different people rushed in and out of the room. Sandeep stood aside, not knowing what to do. He is always so confident and assured, but I remember his helplessness as he questioned the nurse. Then the resident who had been there earlier entered and took control. They put an oxygen mask on me and she would try to get the heart rate up again. I had to get on my hands and knees and they manually pushed the baby back and forth. I was in pain, but I knew it was for my little baby.

That did it: the heart rate came back up and the oxygen mask remained. Everyone breathed easier. I told my husband to inform the others of what had occurred.

Once I had the epidural, Shivani and I watched the contractions on the monitor. We discussed baby names, which Sandeep and I were still debating. He wanted an American name for the baby, since as an immigrant, he found his nick-name Sandy made life simpler. On the other hand, having been raised in the U.S., I wanted to give the baby an Indian name to root her. It may be difficult at first, but people get used to it and it's unique. We had decided to give an Indian first name and American middle name, giving the child the option to choose. My dream was to find a name that was culturally transient.

This would actually break naming traditions. In our region of India, it is customary for the child to use the father's first name as a middle name. This practice helps identify a patriarchal lineage. My middle name was my father's name and it was expected that when I got married I would accept my husband's first name as my middle name. When I grew up, girls had middle names like Marie and Anne. It was awkward to announce my middle name was Harnish. When I got married, I moved my last name Jani into the middle name slot. I definitely wanted my child to have his or her own name. Because we were unable to learn the gender of the baby, we decided we would need two first and two middle names ready for either sex. The name selection included hours of internet surfing, sipping chai lattes at Borders, and finally using spreadsheets to poll our friends. Even at this hour, we had not agreed on spellings of names. Justin Eshaan or Justin Ishaan for a boy. Annika Trisha or Annika Tricia for a girl.

After lunch, everyone was more relaxed and walked in and out of the room. Sandeep found another Indian father-to-be in the hall and came back with updates on his wife's progress. At one point, I realized I needed to use the bathroom, but IV's and wires had me hooked to machines. I called the nurse for assistance to go to the bathroom.

"Now that you had the epidural, you have to stay there," she said.

"No, I'm serious. I really have to go." I insisted. I was quite annoyed. She was professional, but stoic and mechanical. I asked her again in a few minutes.

"Let me see how dilated you are," she said. This annoyed me even more since I really had to go, not deliver. Why is everything about the baby?

"Yep, you're ready to go. But I'm off duty now," she said before she left the room. I was stunned.

On the Day You Were Born

Lisa, the friendly nurse from the previous night, entered and we cheered to see her. She said I was ready to push and called the doctor. The doctor checked as well, and she said it was time. I kept my eyes on Lisa and took my cues from her when to push and let go. My sister looked at her watch and it was 3:00 p.m.

"If we get done by 4:00, we can watch Oprah!" she said.

"Do you think the baby should be watching today's show?" asked one of the nurses. Shivani and the nurses continued chatting about Oprah. I smiled weakly with them.

Sandeep was on my left and held my hand. Aunt Sudha stood next to him. My sister was on my right with my mother next to her. The hospital policy, we were told on the day of our tour, allowed only two people in the delivery room. Here I had four and no one was saying anything.

Like I had done in my Lamaze classes, I closed my eyes and tried to focus on my breathing. I remember my sister telling me "You can do it, do it for the baby." My husband was holding my hand and telling me to push. I grunted and the doctor told me to be quiet.

"Focus your energies on pushing the baby. Don't talk."

"Is anything happening?" I asked.

"Yes, it's coming along great," said the nurse.

"Are you sure?" I asked. I wasn't feeling a thing and this pushing business was getting boring.

"What do you mean, 'Are you sure?' Yes, we're sure! Let's get ready again," the doctor laughed.

We pushed for an hour and I had my eyes closed. Then the contractions became stronger and the pain was unbearable. I cried for my mom, who jumped next to me to hold my hand. Shivani was pushed further on the sideline. The doctor had to do an episiotomy. At this point, my sister began to lose it. She later said it was a combination of the sight of blood, my cries for my mom, and the "snip" she heard. There was more pushing and cheering. I had my eyes closed and tried to do what I was told.

Suddenly I felt a squiggly animal between my legs. I screamed and jumped. I opened my eyes and everybody was cheering and crying, "A girl! A girl!"

They put her on my stomach and I cried, "My baby, oh my baby," over and over. I wanted to kiss her, but through my tears, I could see a bloody mat of dark hair and I was afraid to touch her yet. Even before I could, if I had wanted to, they scooped her away to an alcove for examination.

I saw my husband wipe away tears and hug me. Aunt Sudha was crying. My mother followed the baby with the nurses to an alcove in the room. My sister looked a little pale and I asked her if she was all right. The doctor told her to sit down. As she sat, she fainted into a chair. My mother came to me, dizzy with excitement about the baby, but I told her to look at my sister, slumped in the armchair. My mother shook her shoulder.

"What's wrong with you? Why are you sleeping?"

Shivani looked up drowsily. I told my mother she fainted and she replied, "Humph." She turned to me with the brightest eyes, and said, "She's a beautiful baby. You have to see her."

In the meantime, while my support team was with the baby, I felt alone as the doctor gave me stitches. I wasn't sure if this hurt more than the actual delivery. Someone would come over for a minute or two to make sure I was all right and report on the baby. Then they would scurry back to the alcove. This was just a sign of things yet to come, I told myself.

"What time was she born?" I asked.

"About 15 minutes ago, at 4:02," the nurse reported.

"We can still catch Oprah!" said my sister, perking up.

It is an Indian tradition on the birth of a child to distribute sweets. Aunt Sudha pulled out a pineapple cake that she had made and as it was Valentine's Day, my mother had boxes of chocolates for the staff. Aunt Sudha took out special blankets that she quilted and knitted for the baby. There was a shawl that belonged to Sandeep's grandmother, and she wanted a photograph to send back to India. Aunt Sudha actually left other special "birth" day and Valentine's Day presents she had carried with her at home.

The baby was now Annika Trisha Desai. Annika means *Grace* in Scandinavian and Hebrew and is another name for *Goddess Durga* in Sanskrit. The name Trisha is a derivative of the Sanskrit word for *thirst* or *desire*. We were both confident when we signed the birth certificate that this was it.

That evening, my father, my brother, and Sandeep's brother came to visit us. A banana nut cake was impulsively purchased and we sang "Happy Birthday, Annika." We all made wishes to her on the video camera and made tearful regrets for the family who could not be with us.

That night, I asked that Annika be kept in the nursery, which would allow me to recover. My visitors left and I was alone for the first time. I stole a few moments to jot the events in my journal. I nibbled on my mom's snacks and the banana cake, since the hospital dinner was weak. The nurses would check on me periodically, so continuous sleep was not an option. Plus, I was focused on how to get in and out of bed to use the restroom constantly. I was dealing with hot flashes and shivers due to hormone fluctuations; I thought it was due to the crazy heating system at the hospital until I was told otherwise.

The next morning, I hobbled to the bathroom to wash. The nurse wheeled in the bassinet and said, "Here's your baby." It sounds funny to say it, but I had almost forgotten about her. I had been so caught up in my own body and needs that I had forgotten there was a baby. I started crying. *I had a baby.* She was lying there, all tightly swaddled with her dark eyes darting around.

Who are you, little one? I wanted to ask her. *Are you really mine?* I embraced her and kept staring. My little bird stared back at me with equal intensity.

Every story I read in my parenting magazines said the mother "knew" right away how perfect her baby was. I felt empty. I wasn't sure if this was really right. She had my husband's nose, a short and wide bulbous aperture. She had rosy cheeks and puffy eyes. I don't have rosy cheeks or puffy eyes. She did not look like the baby I thought I would have with my dark eyebrows or a long Jani nose. Last night, my father said he was nonchalant about the pregnancy until he saw her and he fell in love. I felt confused. *What do we do now?* When my sister had asked Annika, "Do you want to go to Mom?" I thought she meant my mother, not me. *Me, a mom?*

Sandeep and Aunt Sudha came in the morning with hot Starbucks lattes. I had eliminated caffeine for nine months and I would splurge now. The coffee seemed more comforting to hold than the tiny baby. My anxiety grew as breastfeeding was uneventful, except for the pain. Every hiccup and poopy diaper made us nervous about our capabilities. We asked the nurse to show us how to change the diaper, bathe her, and buckle her in a car seat. While it seems cliché for new parents, I felt it was true—how could we be allowed to leave with her?

Aunt Sudha returned to Canada on Thursday. We told her to stay one more day, but she insisted we needed quiet time as a family. Then she fluttered away as quickly as she had arrived. When her children called us in the hospital, they were surprised by our happy reports. She truly supported all of us throughout this experience. They conceded that while she may seem light and flippant, when needed, she's a rock.

When we went home on Friday, I played *The Carpenters Greatest Hits* CD. When I was pregnant, I listened to this CD often, hoping Carpenters and Sarah McLachlan would become recognizable lullabies. It was like magic—Annika would fall asleep immediately within the first few notes of "Close to You" or "We've Only Just Begun."

We started wondering whether she was an old hippie in her past life. Annika had a look of wisdom beyond her days. She studied everyone like an old person, trying to understand. She was really an "alert" baby and a "people-person," and I attribute it to the fact that there were so many people in the room when she was born.

It was in the wee hours of the morning that I felt our true bonding experience occur. I was nursing her in bed and caressing her dark hair. The house was quiet. I felt like the whole world was asleep but the two of us. She looked like my husband. I thought of my love for my husband, and I felt a wave of love and recognition towards her. This was it. She's our little girl.

That period of being unfamiliar with each other seems foreign to me now. We are no longer strangers, but a family connected. She's wrapped herself around her father's heart and, of course, he and I are both different people now. We know a new meaning of love on Valentine's Day.

29

At the Threshold

Jamaica Ritcher

There was before: the chicken curry that your papa made because I had a cold, and the movie that we watched about the 20-somethings and their night on the town. Beautifully self-centered, they did everything and nothing at all. As the credits rolled there was his casual remark, marking the reality that our remaining nights like this were few, and my tears with the admission that no, the nights like this were gone.

There was the bursting balloon inside me and astonished nurses—*Did you get a load of her? Smiling and cracking jokes?*—as I waddled round the corner, excited to have a baby, not knowing what that meant for the coming hours: the stick and flow of the IV drip, squeeze of the monitor belt, a red line keeping time with my pain.

There was the searing and wrenching, white knuckles and timid attempts to push, an obstetrician off to the side, absently cracking her knuckles during the pause between contractions, and my psychedelic hospital gown that the next morning was only polka dots. There was the frustration of you, squeezing up and sliding back again, until I began to doubt nature, and what I was meant to do.

Then there is you, finally slipping out into a pair of hands that hand you up, placing you upon me still connected by a cord, belly to belly, now on the other side, and the sound of my breath, stunned inhalations and tears.

And this is the moment I die, my life melting away like the ice chips on my tongue, dissolving into purpose larger than myself, into you and we and the weight of mutual need. This is the moment of fumbling introduction, of love untainted by misspoken words and intentions. An instant, and I become your mother.

Afterword

I was a nosy child. I was about six years old when I riffled through my mother's file cabinet while she was busy somewhere else in the house and, by happy coincidence, found the journal entry she'd written about giving birth. According to my mother, I was "perfect"—I had none of the wrinkly redness of most newborns, no birthmarks, just pure beauty with a head full of dark hair that my mother, like God, pronounced good. That was almost three decades ago, but I never forgot finding and reading that essay. It was clear, from reading her short piece, that giving birth ranked among the best experiences she ever expected to have, that it fulfilled dreams she had had for years, that she was terribly grateful not just to be *a* mother but to be *my* mother. It made me feel terribly loved.

Perhaps that experience, so many years ago, planted a seed that became the impetus for this book. When I discovered that thousands of women post their "birth stories" on the internet every day, that thousands of women read other women's birth stories every day, and that this is a burgeoning market on the world wide web, I remembered my mother's story and I realized that here was a book, a book that could explore this visceral yet extra-worldly experience of giving birth. The majority of men and women in the world have, at one time or another, given birth or supported their partners through that beautiful and terrible experience. Giving birth is a time when one's best dreams and ideas—and worst fears and nightmares—coalesce into a single moment of anticipation. Out of such moments come stories that reach into the deepest place of what it means to be human, what it means to be a spiritual being, what it means to love and be loved.

Ordinary men and women who have participated in this act of giving birth have written the essays collected here. All of the contributors have been transformed by their experiences, changed at some core level of their being, and this is what they try to define in their writing. For some, the experience was what it "should" be—without complication, a joyous event that caught them up in rapture. For others, the experience was everything it "shouldn't" be—resulting in death, or mental health issues, or destruction. Yet all would agree with Pierre Laroche, who writes that watching his wife give birth helped him to understand not only her "story"—that is, "who" she is—but also her body, the parts of her, her "gears"—that is, "what" she is.

The fact that giving birth has become a metaphor for so many of our other experiences suggests its importance as a milestone experience in a person's life, as well as its importance on a grander, more cosmological level for the human race. One of the ways I began to think about giving birth while editing this anthology is that it is one of the most holy acts we can participate in. At its core level, it is completely biological, completely natural; yet is it also fundamentally supernatural, causing us to contemplate all sorts of spiritual mysteries: the nature of life and death, the connection between the spiritual and natural world. Giving birth is a very non-religious, non-spiritual act; yet it is also a very Buddhist, very Christian, very Muslim, very Hindu, very human and very spiritual act. As the Hebrew poet and king, David, wrote in a prayer to his God:

> For you formed my inward parts;
> You covered me in my mother's womb.
> I will praise you,
> For I am fearfully and wonderfully made;
> Marvelous are your works,
> And that my soul knows well.
> —Psalm 139, New King James Version

Jessica Powers, Editor
San Bruno, California
September 2008

Contributor Bios

Ann Angel *is the contributing editor of* Such A Pretty Face, Short Stories about Beauty. *Her biography* Under the Influence, the Life and Times of Janis Joplin *will be released by Abrams/Amulet in 2009.*

Elisabeth Aron *is an OB/GYN and the author of* Pregnancy Dos and Don'ts: the Smart Woman's A-Z Pocket Companion for a Safe and Sound Pregnancy.

Sarah Briggs *teaches violin at Amherst and Smith Colleges and is a member of the Florence Piano Trio. Her son, Stone, came as a late-in-life delight.*

Tina Cassidy *is a journalist and author of* Birth: The Surprising History of How We Are Born. *She lives in Boston with her husband and two sons.*

Kelley Cunningham *is a part-time fine artist and illustrator, a weekend humor writer, a full-time art director in children's publishing, and the proud mom of three wonderful boys. She lives in Pennsylvania with her family. She wishes there were more hours in the day to paint, read, and enjoy her kids.*

Karen Deaver *writes, publishes, and teaches writing as much as she can while remaining mindful of her two sons' perfect youth. She and her family live in New Jersey.*

Ashini J. Desai *earned a B.A. in English and an M.S. in Information Science, balancing poetry, project management, and motherhood. She writes for South Asian websites, as well as her own site (www.ashinid.blogspot.com),* Philadelphia Poets, *and* Thema. *She and her family live in Pennsylvania.*

Martin Edwards *is a creative journeyman, making a living as a photographer, filmmaker and writer. He lives in Berkeley with his wife and sons.*

Ariel Gore *is the editor-publisher of* Hip Mama *and the author of several books, including her latest,* How to Become a Famous Writer Before You're Dead: Your Words in Print and Your Name in Lights. *Her blog is www.arielgore.com.*

Joan Labbe *lives near Boston with her husband, her daughter Aline and her son Nicky. Nicky was born with midwives in attendance and came out way too fast for his mama to think he could possibly get stuck. Joan continues to work on* Opening to life.

Pierre Laroche *is a professor in the department of English & Communication at Doña Ana Community College in Las Cruces, New Mexico, where he lives with his wife and two sons.*

Erin Lassiter *lives in San Diego, California with her partner and her two children. She works as a freelance writer, creating curriculum materials for teachers and elementary school students, and as a mosaic artist.*

Annalysa Lovos's *articles have appeared in* Mothering, The Sun, *and* New Mobility, *and she is currently working on her first book. She and her husband Dave, a musician and luthier, and Sage make their home in northwestern Montana's Flathead Valley.*

Noemi Martinez *is a community activist, poet, writer and single mother. She has been writing the zine* Hermana, Resist *for seven years and is the unofficial "zine queen."*

Frederica Mathewes-Green *is the author of eight books, including* Facing East: A Pilgrim's Journey into the Mysteries of Orthodoxy. *She lives in Baltimore, Maryland with her husband, the Reverend Gregory Mathewes-Green.*

Jennifer Mattern *is a playwright and freelance writer based in western Massachusetts. Her award-winning blog on parenting,* Breed 'Em and Weep, *can be read at www. breedemandweep.com.*

Jeannette Monsivais-Ruiter *teaches French, Spanish, and Speech at Loretto Academy in El Paso. She lives in El Paso with her husband David and daughter Catherine.*

Amy Parker *lives in Maryland in the Washington D.C. Suburbs. She and her husband Craig live with their 7-year-old twins and a 2 1/2-year-old son, whom she actually got to carry! After everything she and her husband went through with the twins, being able to get pregnant was a dream come true. Amy continues to live each day as a stay-at-home mom, learning new lessons, and hopefully teaching some lessons along the way.*

William Pierce's *fiction and essays have appeared in* American Literary Review, The Writer's Chronicle, The Cincinnati Review, *and elsewhere. He also writes a series of essays for* AGNI *entitled "Crucibles." From 1998 to 2004, he was a stay-at-home dad. Now his children, a ten-year-old girl and seven-year-old boy, look after him.*

Sabrina Porterfield *is the 40-year-old mother of twins and lives with her wife in Finland. When she isn't chasing the twins around, she systematically attempts to brainwash a select group of women online to trade warm weather for positive social policies, decent health care, and naked firemen.*

Jessica Powers *writes for young adults under the name J.L. Powers. Her novel,* The Confessional, *was published by Knopf in 2007. Catalyst Book Press is her company, which she started in 2007.* Labor Pains and Birth Stories *is the press's second book.*

Tania Pryputniewicz *is a graduate of the Iowa Writers Workshop. Her cover art, "Invisible Helpers," was drawn, carved and rolled out three weeks before the birth of her first child. She lives in the California redwoods with her husband and three children, where she writes on Fridays and attempts to keep her blog (www.poetrymom.blogspot.com) current while caring for her family.*

Diana M. Raab, *R.N., MFA, is widely published in national magazines. She teaches writing at the UCLA Extension Writers' Program. Her book,* Your High-Risk Pregnancy: A Practical and Supportive Guide *is forthcoming in 2009. The book is newly updated and celebrates its 25th anniversary with a preface by Dr. Errol Norwitz. For more information on her other books, visit her website: www.dianaraab.com.*

Michelle Richards *is a freelance writer and Assistant Professor of English in South Florida.*

Jamaica Ritcher's *creative nonfiction has appeared in the online journal* Literary Mama, *on National Public Radio's* Day to Day, *and in* This I Believe: the Personal Philosophies of Remarkable Men and Women *(Henry Holt, 2006). She lives with her husband and two children in Moscow, Idaho.*

Pam Rowen-Herzog *lives in New Mexico with her husband and three boys. Her life is themed around honoring rhythms and rituals, with a strong focus on the emerging Albuquerque Waldorf community and school.*

Melissa Shook *was a documentary photographer, but is now concentrating on video and writing. She has recently retired from the University of Massachusetts at Boston, but still teaches photography part-time. Her website is www.MelissaShook.com.*

Kiersten Forasté Shue *met her husband while living in Taiwan. They settled down in Charlottesville, Virginia, where she now works as a Pilates instructor, freelance writer, and mom. Jett Alexander Shue continues to live up to his speedy name.*

Carmen Gimenez Smith *teaches Creative Writing at New Mexico State University and is the publisher of the small literary press Noemi Press.*

Georgia Tiffany *has received a Washington Commission for the Humanities Grant and a National Endowment for the Arts Grant. Her own writing has won awards and appeared in anthologies and in over 50 different national and international magazines and journals. Her recent chapbook,* Cut from the Score, *was published by Night Owl Press. She teaches and writes in Moscow, Idaho.*

Anne Winterich *has taught high-school English and ESL, but currently volunteers in her daughters' schools and activities. Her poetry has been published in several anthologies including* Words-Myth.

Other Books from Catalyst Book Press

Ken Waldman

Are You Famous? Touring America with Alaska's Fiddling Poet.

Price $15.00 ISBN 978-0-980208-10-8

Ken Waldman has toured throughout North America as Alaska's Fiddling Poet since 1995. He is the author of six poetry collections and has released seven CDs. This, his first book of prose, is part memoir, part travel notes, and part artist how-to. A Blue Highways for 2009.

A great read. For those who've wondered what it's like to live a life on the road in pursuit of one's passion, here's your book. Those who already know what it's like can point and say, "It's like this." —Jeff Talmadge, CoraZong Records recording artist, internationally touring singer/songwriter.

Call for Submissions

Catalyst Book Press is seeking literary essays telling personal stories related to fertility. Planned anthologies in late 2009 and early 2010 include an anthology of stories about miscarriage and another anthology of personal stories about adoption, open adoption, birth parent connections, the adoption triad, and unification with children after closed adoption for an anthology for and about birth parents. Future anthologies include stories about postpartum depression, stories about abortion, stories about large families, stories of infertility, stories about giving birth at home, and stories by midwives. Updated guidelines are available at www. catalystbookpress.com.

Printed in the United States
130650LV00003B/163-225/P